The Hidden Power of Castor Oil: Nature's Ultimate Elixir Revealed

Unlock Ancient Holistic Secrets to
Reduce Inflammation, Boost Wellness,
and Rediscover Your Glow with
Practical Everyday Tips

Barbara Harris

© Copyright 2025 - All rights reserved.

The contents of this book may not be reproduced, duplicated, or transmitted without direct written permission from the author. Unauthorized use or distribution is strictly prohibited.

Disclaimer Notice

This book was written with assistance from AI tools and is intended for educational and entertainment purposes only. The information provided is based on publicly available sources and does not constitute legal, financial, medical, or professional advice.

While every effort has been made to ensure accuracy, no warranties of any kind are expressed or implied. The author and publisher disclaim all responsibility for any errors, omissions, or inaccuracies and are not liable for any direct or indirect losses resulting from the use of this information.

Readers are encouraged to consult licensed professionals before applying any techniques or recommendations outlined in this book. The content is not a substitute for expert guidance.

By reading this book, you agree that the author and publisher bear no liability for any damages, losses, or consequences incurred as a result of the use or misuse of the content.

To illustrate key concepts and ideas for educational purposes, some stories and case studies in this book have been adapted or created. They may draw from a blend of real-life examples or be entirely fictional to effectively convey the intended message

Copyright © 2025 by JAD Publishing Ltd

Table of Contents

Introduction

Chapter 1: Unveiling Castor Oil's Historical Legacy
1.1 From Ancient Egypt to Modern Day: The Timeless Journey of Castor Oil
1.2 Traditional Remedies: Castor Oil in Ayurvedic Practices
1.3 Castor Oil in Ancient Chinese Medicine: A Heritage of Healing
1.4 The African Connection: Castor Oil in Tribal Medicine
1.5 Mediterranean Traditions: Castor Oil's Role in Classic Health Practices

Chapter 2: The Science Behind Castor Oil's Efficacy
2.1 Castor Oil and Skin Health: A Scientific Approach
2.2 The Molecular Magic: How Castor Oil Boosts Immunity
2.3 Hair Growth Unveiled: Science Behind Castor Oil's Effectiveness
2.4 Castor Oil and Digestive Health: A Look at the Science

Chapter 3: Selecting and Storing Authentic Castor Oil
3.1 Certifications and Quality: Ensuring Authenticity
3.2 Storage Solutions: Preserving Potency and Freshness

3.3 Recognizing Adulterated Products: Red Flags to Watch For

Chapter 4: Practical Applications for Health and Wellness
4.1 Boosting Immunity: Daily Rituals with Castor Oil
4.2 Natural Pain Relief: Castor Oil for Muscle and Joint Comfort
4.3 Enhancing Digestion: Recipes and Techniques
4.4 Castor Oil Packs: A Step-by-Step Guide for Internal Healing
4.5 Detoxifying the Body: Integrating Castor Oil into Cleansing Practices

Chapter 5: Beauty and Personal Care with Castor Oil
5.1 DIY Skincare: Radiant Skin with Castor Oil
5.2 Luscious Locks: Hair Treatment Recipes
5.3 Castor Oil in Anti-Aging Regimens: Natural Youthfulness
5.4 Nail and Cuticle Care: Strengthening with Castor Oil
5.5 Natural Makeup Remover: A Gentle Alternative

Chapter 6: Holistic Health and Lifestyle Integration
6.1 Incorporating Castor Oil into Yoga and Meditation Practices
6.2 Balancing Chakras: Energetic Uses of Castor Oil
6.3 Castor Oil in Aromatherapy: Blends for Mindfulness
6.4 Creating Daily Rituals: Mindful Living with Castor Oil

Chapter 7: Addressing Common Concerns and Missteps
7.1 Safe Use Guidelines: Avoiding Common Pitfalls
7.2 Dosage and Application: Getting It Right Every Time
7.3 Combining Castor Oil with Other Natural Remedies
7.4 Recognizing and Managing Adverse Reactions

Chapter 8: Sustainability and Environmental Impact

8.1 Castor Oil and Environmental Stewardship
8.2 The Role of Castor Oil in Zero Waste Living
8.3 Green Beauty: Eco-Conscious Personal Care Choices

Chapter 9: Exploring Unique and Niche Uses
9.1 Castor Oil in Pet Care: Benefits and Precautions
9.2 Industrial Insights: Non-Toxic Household Solutions
9.3 Artistic Applications: Using Castor Oil in Creative Projects
9.4 Castor Oil in Traditional Crafts: Reviving Old Techniques

Chapter 10: Personal Stories and Expert Insights
10.1 Expert Interviews: Insights from Natural Health Practitioners
10.2 Testimonials: Real-Life Benefits and Experiences
10.3 Insider Tips: Maximizing Castor Oil Benefits
10.4 The Future of Castor Oil: Trends and Innovations
10.5 Interactive Experience: Enhancing Learning with QR Codes
10.6 Beyond Borders: Castor Oil's Global Impact
10.7 Your Wellness Journey: Embracing Castor Oil for Life

Conclusion

The Hidden Power Of Castor Oil

References

Introduction

In a small village on the banks of the Nile thousands of years ago, people discovered a curious oil. This oil came from the seeds of the castor plant. It was thick, golden, and had a peculiar scent. Villagers quickly found that it could soothe aches, heal wounds, and even nurture the skin. This was the beginning of castor oil's long journey as a natural remedy. It has traveled through time, finding its place in both ancient and modern medicine cabinets. Today, castor oil remains a versatile elixir, bridging the wisdom of our ancestors with contemporary science.

The purpose of this book is to guide you in rediscovering the practical benefits of castor oil. It aims to show how ancient wisdom can seamlessly blend into modern life. By the end of this journey, you will see how this simple oil can enhance your health, beauty, and overall well-being. The pages ahead will offer a practical guide to incorporating this age-old remedy into your daily routine.

My passion for natural remedies began years ago. I remember my grandmother using castor oil for nearly everything—from her aching joints to her glowing skin. Watching her, I developed a keen interest in understanding how nature's gifts could support our health. This personal journey has fueled my dedication to helping others explore and benefit from the bounty of natural solutions, with castor oil being a particular focus.

What makes castor oil unique among natural oils? The secret lies in its composition. It is rich in ricinoleic acid, a rare fatty acid that holds the key to its various benefits. This acid gives castor oil its anti-inflammatory, antimicrobial, and moisturizing properties. It can soothe the skin, relieve pain, and even promote hair growth. Few other oils can boast such a wide range of uses.

This book is an invitation to embark on a journey of discovery. You will find a holistic approach that combines historical insights, scientific research, and practical applications. Each chapter offers a new perspective on how castor oil can be used in your life. I encourage you to read with an open mind and a willingness to experiment with what you learn.

The structure of this book is straightforward. We start with the historical uses of castor oil, tracing its journey through time. Next, we explore the scientific insights that explain why this oil is effective. Following that, you will find practical applications, including recipes and techniques that you can try at home. Personal stories and experiences are woven throughout, providing real-life examples of castor oil's impact.

I want to assure you that the information in this book is well-researched and reliable. I have consulted with experts and delved into numerous studies to bring you accurate and trustworthy content. My goal is to provide you with a comprehensive understanding of how castor oil can benefit you.

As you read, I encourage you to engage actively with the content. Try the recipes and techniques. Share your experiences and insights. This book is not just informational; it is designed to be interactive and transformative. Your journey with castor oil is personal and unique, and I hope it brings you new insights and benefits.

I would like to close this introduction with a thought: Embracing natural solutions like castor oil is not just about looking to the past. It is about finding balance in the present and nurturing a future of well-being. As you turn the pages, remember that integrating ancient wisdom into your modern lifestyle is a powerful way to achieve health and harmony. Let this book be your guide in that journey.

Chapter 1
Unveiling Castor Oil's Historical Legacy

In the warm glow of a flickering torch, an ancient Egyptian embalmer worked meticulously, surrounded by an array of mysterious substances. Among them was a humble oil, derived from the seeds of the castor plant. This oil, with its distinct aroma and viscous texture, held within it secrets that transcended time. As the embalmers prepared the departed for their journey to the afterlife, castor oil played a crucial role. It was not just a tool of preservation but a symbol of protection and respect for the deceased. The ancient Egyptians believed that preserving the body was essential for the soul's eternal rest, and castor oil was a key ingredient in this sacred ritual. This practice was not only about mummification but also about the belief in continuity and the seamless transition between life and death. As we begin our exploration of castor oil's historical legacy, we will uncover how this simple oil became an integral part of both ancient and modern lives.

1.1 From Ancient Egypt to Modern Day: The Timeless Journey of Castor Oil

Castor oil's journey begins in the golden sands of Ancient Egypt, where it was a staple in both health and beauty rituals. Egyptians revered it not only for its medicinal properties but also for its role in preserving the dead. The oil was used in embalming processes, a practice reflecting the Egyptians' profound belief in the afterlife. According to recent biochemical analyses, this oil, among other substances, was applied to the head and other body parts to prevent bacterial growth and maintain the body's integrity [1] The famed queen Cleopatra is said to have used castor oil to enhance her beauty, particularly for her eyes, demonstrating its early use in cosmetics. Hieroglyphs and archaeological findings further cement castor oil's place in Egyptian culture, showcasing its importance in rituals and daily life.

As centuries passed, castor oil traversed through empires, carried along trade routes that spanned continents. The oil found new homes in the bustling markets of Rome, the bazaars of Persia, and the bustling ports of India. Each culture adapted it to their needs, incorporating it into their own healing and beauty practices. The Industrial Revolution marked another turning point in castor oil's history. With advancements in production, it became more accessible, finding its way into factories as a lubricant and in households as a remedy for common ailments. This period of industrialization not only expanded castor oil's applications but also solidified its presence in the global market.

---

1. *The Surprising Substances Ancient Egyptians Used to ...* https://www.smithsonianmag.com/smart-news/the-surprising-substances-ancient-egyptians-used-to-mummify-the-dead-180981568/

Throughout history, castor oil maintained its place in traditional medicine across various cultures. In India, it became a cornerstone of Ayurvedic medicine, used for its anti-inflammatory and detoxifying properties. In Africa, it was integrated into tribal rituals and healing practices, showcasing its versatility. As societies evolved, so too did castor oil's applications. Modern health practices have integrated it into skincare products and holistic wellness routines, highlighting its enduring relevance. Scientific studies today validate many of the traditional uses of castor oil, confirming its efficacy as an anti-inflammatory and antimicrobial agent.

Castor oil remains a potent symbol of nature's ability to provide solutions that transcend time. Its versatility and effectiveness continue to inspire confidence in its use, from ancient rituals to modern wellness practices.

1.2 Traditional Remedies: Castor Oil in Ayurvedic Practices

In the ancient practice of Ayurveda throughout India and Nepal, castor oil holds a revered place and is often described as the science of life. Known as Gandharvahasta Taila, castor oil is celebrated for its ability to restore balance within the body. Ayurveda, with its rich tapestry of healing, aims to balance the doshas (the fundamental principles)—Vata, Pitta, and Kapha—which are the elemental forces believed to govern our physiological and psychological functions. Castor oil is particularly effective in addressing Vata imbalances, which are associated with qualities like dryness and coldness, leading to conditions such as joint pain or anxiety. Through its warming and lubricating properties, castor oil soothes these imbalances, bringing relief and promoting harmony within the body.

One of the principal roles of castor oil in Ayurveda is in purification and detoxification rituals, known as Panchakarma. This process is not merely about physical cleansing but also about purifying the mind and spirit. Castor oil is utilized in these rituals to gently cleanse the digestive tract, removing toxins and impurities. It is a key component in Virechana therapy, which involves purging to eliminate excess Pitta from the body. This internal cleansing is said to not only improve physical health but also enhance mental clarity, paving the way for a more balanced state of being.

Ayurvedic massage techniques, or Abhyanga, often include castor oil due to its ability to penetrate deeply into the tissues. The oil is warmed and applied with rhythmic strokes to stimulate circulation, ease muscle tension, and calm the nervous system. This practice not only nourishes the skin but also roots the mind, offering a profound sense of relaxation. Such massages are part of daily routines for many, aiming to rejuvenate the body and mind, and they can be adapted to address specific health concerns, such as arthritis or stress.

The holistic benefits of castor oil in Ayurveda extend beyond physical health. It is believed to foster mental clarity and emotional stability. Regular use of castor oil in Ayurvedic practices is said to reduce stress and promote a peaceful mind. This is not just through its physical effects but also through the meditative quality of the rituals themselves. The act of applying the oil, taking time for oneself, and engaging in mindful practices can be deeply therapeutic. This integration of mind, body, and spirit is at the core of Ayurveda, making castor oil a valuable ally in achieving holistic well-being.

The preservation and transmission of these practices have been central to their endurance. Oral traditions, passed down through generations, have kept the knowledge of Ayurvedic remedies alive. Texts like the *Charaka Samhita* document these practices, providing a written record that has guided countless practitioners. This rich tradition has not only survived but thrived, influencing modern holistic health movements worldwide. The principles of Ayurveda, with castor oil as a staple, have found their way into contemporary wellness practices, offering natural solutions in an increasingly synthetic world.

Today, as people seek alternatives to conventional medicine, the ancient wisdom of Ayurveda finds new relevance. Castor oil, with its myriad uses, stands out as a testament to the enduring power of nature. Its integration into modern lifestyles, whether through detoxification, massage, or daily rituals, speaks to its versatility and effectiveness. This ancient oil continues to support those who turn to it, embodying a timeless tradition of healing and balance.

1.3 Castor Oil in Ancient Chinese Medicine: A Heritage of Healing

Traditional Chinese Medicine (TCM) presents a holistic view of health, deeply rooted in the balance of Yin and Yang. This philosophy sees the body as a microcosm of the universe, where harmony and balance are essential for well-being. Within this framework, castor oil found its niche, valued for its ability to harmonize the body's energies. In TCM, the balance of Yin (passive energy) and Yang (active energy) is crucial, and disruptions in this balance often lead to illness. Castor oil, with its warming properties, is used to invigorate Yang energy, promoting a sense of balance and vitality. This oil's inclusion in meridian therapy—a practice involving the stimulation of specific points on the body—demonstrates its importance. By applying castor oil to these points, practitioners aim to enhance the flow of Qi, the life force energy, through the body's meridians, alleviating blockages and restoring health.

In the realm of practical applications, castor oil serves various roles within TCM. One of its prominent uses is in the form of castor oil packs, which are applied to alleviate muscle tension and promote relaxation. These packs, warmed and placed on areas of discomfort, work by enhancing circulation and soothing inflamed tissues. For digestive health, castor oil is employed to gently stimulate the digestive system, addressing issues such as constipation or bloating. Its effectiveness in digestive remedies lies in its ability to stimulate peristalsis, the wave-like contractions of the intestines. Furthermore, for those seeking to balance their Qi, castor oil proves beneficial in skin treatments. By applying it topically, it is believed to harmonize the skin's energy, addressing imbalances that manifest as skin conditions.

In TCM, castor oil is often combined with other herbs to create powerful formulations. The synergy between castor oil and herbs like ginger and licorice root is a prime example. Ginger, known for its warming properties, complements castor oil in relieving cold-induced ailments, while licorice root enhances its anti-inflammatory effects. This combination is frequently used in poultices, a type of herbal compress applied to the skin to draw out impurities and reduce inflammation. These mixtures exemplify the integrative nature of TCM, where the whole is greater than the sum of its parts. By enhancing the efficacy of poultices, castor oil amplifies the healing potential of herbal remedies, making it an indispensable component in TCM formulations.

The historical documentation of castor oil in TCM is rich and varied. Ancient texts like the *Compendium of Materia Medica (Bencao Gangmu)*, a comprehensive encyclopedia of Chinese herbal medicine, provide detailed accounts of its uses. Written by Li Shizhen in the 16th century, this text describes the properties and applications of castor oil, underscoring its significance in Chinese medicine. Historical case studies and anecdotal evidence further illuminate its role, offering glimpses into how castor oil was used in everyday life. These accounts reveal a deep understanding of its therapeutic potential, passed down through generations of practitioners. Such documentation not only cements castor oil's place in TCM but also highlights its enduring relevance in traditional healing practices.

The integration of castor oil into TCM serves as a testament to its versatility and efficacy. Its ability to balance energies, relieve ailments, and complement herbal therapies makes it a valuable tool in the TCM practitioner's arsenal. The rich history and continued use of castor oil in TCM reflect a profound respect for nature's gifts and a commitment to holistic health. As we continue to explore the diverse applications of castor oil, we uncover layers of wisdom that connect us to ancient traditions while offering practical solutions for modern health challenges.

1.4 The African Connection: Castor Oil in Tribal Medicine

In the vast and varied landscapes of Africa, castor oil has woven itself into the cultural and medicinal tapestry of many tribes. Among the Himba people of Namibia, castor oil is a cherished component of hair care rituals. The Himba, known for their distinctive hairstyles and vibrant red ochre body paint, utilize castor oil to nourish and protect their hair amidst the harsh desert climate. Women meticulously apply castor oil mixed with red ochre to their braids, not only to preserve moisture but also to symbolize beauty and cultural identity. This ritual is more than cosmetic; it is a testament to the resilience and ingenuity of traditional practices, where castor oil stands as a guardian of heritage and identity in the face of environmental challenges.

Beyond hair care, castor oil plays a pivotal role in the spiritual and healing ceremonies of numerous African tribes. In these communities, health and spirituality are deeply intertwined, with castor oil often serving as a conduit for cleansing and renewal. During ceremonies aimed at spiritual purification, healers use castor oil to anoint participants, believing that its properties can cleanse the spirit and protect against negative energies. This practice reflects a broader worldview where physical and spiritual health are inseparable and castor oil acts as a bridge between the corporeal and the ethereal.

The socio-cultural significance of castor oil extends far beyond its practical uses. In many African societies, it symbolizes unity and community health. Tribal ceremonies where castor oil is used often involve communal participation, reinforcing social bonds and collective identity. In these gatherings, castor oil is not just a remedy; it is a symbol of shared heritage and communal resilience. It plays a role in rites of passage, healing rituals, and celebrations, marking it as a vital component of cultural continuity.

The use of castor oil in Africa did not remain isolated. The trans-Saharan trade routes facilitated the exchange of goods and ideas, including medicinal knowledge. Castor oil became a commodity of interest, exchanged not just for its practical benefits but also for the cultural insights it carried. African uses of castor oil influenced, and were influenced by, other cultures along these trade routes. This exchange enriched the collective understanding of its properties, leading to a cross-continental appreciation of its benefits. Through these interactions, castor oil was woven into the broader narrative of global medicinal practices, influencing and being influenced by the diverse cultures it touched.

Efforts to preserve the traditional knowledge surrounding castor oil continue today, as ethnobotanists and historians work to document these practices. Oral histories provide a rich tapestry of stories, detailing the ways castor oil has been used and adapted over generations. These stories are complemented by ethnobotanical studies that seek to understand the scientific basis of traditional uses, validating and preserving the wisdom of the past. This book not only honors the cultural heritage of African tribes but also ensures that the legacy of castor oil continues to inspire future generations. In modern times, these efforts are crucial in maintaining the connection between traditional practices and contemporary applications, allowing castor oil to remain a vibrant part of both cultural identity and practical health solutions.

1.5 Mediterranean Traditions: Castor Oil's Role in Classic Health Practices

In the sun-drenched lands of ancient Greece and Rome, health and wellness were not just aspects of life but pillars of culture. The Greeks, with their profound respect for balance and harmony, embraced the principles of Hippocratic medicine. Hippocrates, often called the "Father of Medicine," laid the groundwork for a system that emphasized natural healing and the body's ability to restore itself. Within this framework, castor oil found its place as a valuable therapeutic agent. The Greeks understood the importance of maintaining the body's equilibrium and used various natural substances, including castor oil, to achieve this. Meanwhile, the Romans, renowned for their opulent bathhouses and indulgent lifestyle, integrated castor oil into their elaborate bathing rituals. These bathhouses were not only places of cleanliness but also centers of social life and relaxation, where castor oil was used as an emollient to soften skin and as a restorative to soothe the body after the stresses of daily life.

In daily life, castor oil was an indispensable element in both Greek and Roman societies. It served multiple purposes, from personal care to medicinal applications. As a skin emollient, it provided moisture and protection, making it a staple in beauty routines. The oil's rich, viscous nature allowed it to penetrate deeply, nourishing and revitalizing the skin, much like the olive oil that was so cherished in the region.

For hair, castor oil's conditioning properties helped maintain luster and strength, proving its worth as a natural treatment. Additionally, its role as a purgative was well recognized. The oil's ability to stimulate digestion and cleanse the system made it a favored remedy for digestive ailments, aligning with the Mediterranean focus on diet and gut health.

The Mediterranean diet, celebrated for its emphasis on whole foods and healthy fats, seamlessly integrated castor oil into its regimen. While olive oil was the predominant fat, castor oil found its niche in specific applications. It was used sparingly in cooking, valued for its unique properties and medicinal benefits. Castor oil complemented other oils, enhancing the nutritional profile of meals and supporting digestive health. The synergy between castor oil and olive oil, both rich in beneficial fatty acids, exemplifies the Mediterranean approach to health: simple, natural ingredients working together to nourish and heal. This integration underscores the Mediterranean belief in the power of food as medicine, a philosophy that continues to influence modern dietary practices.

Archaeological evidence and ancient texts provide a window into the historical use of castor oil in the Mediterranean. Pedanius Dioscorides, a Greek physician and botanist, documented the properties of castor oil in his seminal work, *Materia Medica*, a comprehensive catalog of medicinal plants and their uses. His writings offer detailed insights into the oil's applications, underscoring its significance in ancient medicine. Excavations of Roman sites have uncovered amphorae and containers that once held castor oil, testifying to its widespread use. These findings, coupled with literary references, paint a vivid picture of castor oil's role in the daily and medicinal life of Mediterranean civilizations. They reveal a culture that valued natural remedies and understood the therapeutic potential of this versatile oil.

The Mediterranean tradition of using castor oil reflects a broader wisdom that harmonizes with nature's rhythms. It highlights an ancient understanding of health that resonates with contemporary values, where simplicity and efficacy are prized. As we reflect on these practices, we find ourselves connected to a lineage of knowledge that transcends time, offering lessons in balance and well-being. The enduring legacy of castor oil in Mediterranean health practices not only enriches our understanding of ancient cultures but also inspires us to embrace natural solutions in our own lives. The journey of castor oil, from the ancient Mediterranean to modern times, is a testament to its timeless relevance and the enduring power of nature's gifts.

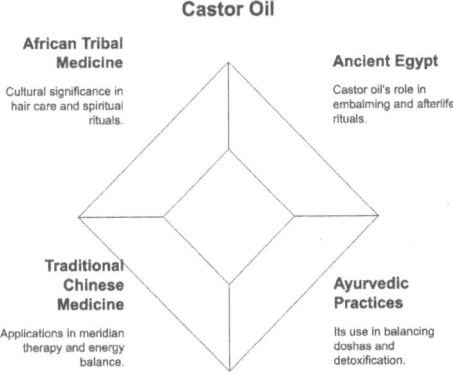

Chapter 2
The Science Behind Castor Oil's Efficacy

Imagine a tiny molecule with the power to influence your health and well-being. This is ricinoleic acid, the key component in castor oil, responsible for many of its celebrated benefits. Found in the seeds of the Ricinus communis plant, ricinoleic acid comprises about 90% of the oil's composition [2]. Its unique structure is what makes castor oil so effective. Ricinoleic acid is an 18-carbon fatty acid with a distinctive architecture. It features a hydroxyl group strategically positioned at the 12th carbon and an unsaturated bond nestled between the 9th and 10th carbon. This configuration is not just a structural curiosity; it gives ricinoleic acid its remarkable properties. The hydroxyl group, in particular, enhances the fatty acid's polarity, making it a potent agent for skin penetration and moisture retention. The unsaturated bond, meanwhile, contributes to the fluidity and flexibility of the molecule, allowing it to interact effectively with biological membranes.

The biological activities of ricinoleic acid are as fascinating as its structure. It is renowned for its anti-inflammatory properties, which help reduce swelling and pain. This makes it a popular choice for relieving conditions such as arthritis and muscle aches. When applied to the skin, ricinoleic acid penetrates the layers, influencing the production of prostaglandins, which are compounds that regulate inflammation in the body. By modulating these pathways, ricinoleic acid can significantly reduce inflammation, providing relief from discomfort. Moreover, its antimicrobial activity adds another layer of protection, guarding against bacteria and fungi. This makes castor oil an effective treatment for minor skin infections and irritations, such as ringworm and dermatitis (SOURCE 3). The antimicrobial action is largely due to ricinoleic acid's ability to disrupt the cell membranes of pathogens, inhibiting their growth and proliferation.

The high viscosity of castor oil, attributed to ricinoleic acid, is another factor that sets it apart from other oils. This thickness is not merely a textural characteristic but plays a crucial role in its application and effectiveness. When you apply castor oil to the skin, its viscous nature allows it to form a protective barrier, sealing in moisture and preventing dehydration. This makes it an excellent emollient for dry or chapped skin, offering long-lasting hydration. The thick consistency also ensures that when used in massage or topical treatments, the oil stays in place, allowing for prolonged interaction with the skin. This is particularly beneficial in therapeutic applications, where sustained contact can enhance the oil's effects, such as in soothing sore muscles or calming irritated skin.

Ricinoleic acid's contribution to castor oil's therapeutic effects extends to pain relief and skin irritation reduction. The fatty acid's structure enables it to penetrate deeply into the skin, reaching the affected areas more effectively than many other topical agents. This deep penetration allows ricinoleic acid to influence the underlying tissues, providing relief from pain and reducing irritation. Its action on prostaglandin production not only alleviates pain but also helps soothe the skin, calming inflammation and promoting healing. These properties make castor oil a versatile tool in managing a range of conditions, from joint pain to eczema.

To better understand how ricinoleic acid works, visualize its structure. Imagine a long chain with a single kink, representing the unsaturated bond, and a small hook, the hydroxyl group, hanging at the 12th carbon. This unique configuration is what sets ricinoleic acid apart, enabling it to interact with the body in ways that other fatty acids cannot. As you explore the uses of castor oil, remember that this tiny molecule is at the heart of its many benefits. Whether you're applying it to soothe an achy joint or using it to moisturize dry skin, ricinoleic acid is working to provide relief and support your health.

2.1 Castor Oil and Skin Health: A Scientific Approach

Start with a small bottle in your hand, filled with a golden liquid. This is castor oil, and it's ready to transform your skin. Its emollient properties create a shield on the skin's surface, locking in moisture and preventing it from escaping. This effect is known as an occlusive barrier, a feature that distinguishes castor oil from lighter oils. Where other oils might evaporate quickly, castor oil stays, offering lasting hydration that softens and smooths even the driest skin. Compare this to coconut or jojoba oil, which are also popular for their moisturizing effects but don't provide the same level of prolonged protection. Castor oil's thickness, while sometimes seen as a drawback, is actually its strength in retaining moisture, making your skin feel supple and nourished.

Beyond just moisture retention, castor oil plays a vital role in enhancing the skin barrier function, an essential aspect of maintaining healthy skin. The skin barrier, primarily composed of lipids in the stratum corneum, acts as a defense against environmental aggressors and prevents water loss. Castor oil supports this barrier by replenishing and repairing these lipid structures, creating a more resilient shield. This is crucial in reducing trans-epidermal water loss (TEWL), which can lead to dehydration and irritation if unchecked. By reinforcing the skin's natural defenses, castor oil not only hydrates but also strengthens, resulting in a complexion that is not only visibly healthier but also better equipped to face the elements. This repair process is akin to patching a leaky roof, where every drop of oil contributes to a more secure and stable structure.

The antimicrobial effects of castor oil extend its benefits beyond hydration and barrier support. Scientific studies have shown that castor oil is effective against common skin pathogens, including bacteria and fungi. This makes it an excellent choice for treating conditions such as acne and dermatitis. In these cases, the oil's ability to penetrate the skin and disrupt microbial activity helps clear infections and soothe inflammation. By targeting the root cause of these skin issues, castor oil offers a natural remedy that can reduce reliance on harsher chemical treatments. Its antimicrobial properties are like having a tiny army of protectors on your skin, ready to ward off any unwelcome invaders that threaten its health.

Wound healing is another area where castor oil shines. It promotes collagen synthesis, a key process in skin regeneration and repair. Collagen, a protein that provides structure and strength to the skin, is crucial for closing wounds and restoring normal skin texture. By boosting collagen production, castor oil accelerates the healing process, allowing wounds to close more quickly and effectively. This is supported by case studies showing faster wound closure rates in those who use castor oil as part of their treatment regimen. Imagine a cut on your hand; with castor oil, the healing process is not only quicker but also results in smoother, less noticeable scars. This ability to enhance recovery makes castor oil a go-to choice for those seeking natural, effective solutions for skin injuries.

As you explore the benefits of castor oil for skin health, consider how you might incorporate it into your daily routine. Whether as a hydrating treatment for dry patches, a protective layer against environmental damage, or a healing agent for minor cuts and abrasions, castor oil offers a multifaceted approach to skincare. Its unique properties, supported by scientific research, make it a valuable addition to any skincare regimen, providing a natural alternative that works with your body's own processes to promote health and beauty.

2.2 The Molecular Magic: How Castor Oil Boosts Immunity

Castor oil, often seen as a humble household remedy, holds a profound influence on your immune system. At the heart of its immune-boosting power is its ability to stimulate lymphatic function. The lymphatic system, a vital part of your body's defense mechanism, helps maintain fluid balance and filters out harmful substances. Castor oil enhances lymphatic drainage, which is crucial for reducing lymphatic congestion. This is particularly important as congested lymph nodes can lead to swelling and discomfort, hindering your body's ability to fight off infections. By promoting better lymph flow, castor oil assists in detoxifying the body, allowing it to efficiently remove cellular waste and excess fluids. This cleansing action not only boosts your immune system but also contributes to a general sense of well-being.

Another fascinating aspect of castor oil is its impact on macrophages, the white blood cells that play a key role in engulfing and digesting cellular debris and pathogens. Castor oil's stimulation of these cells enhances their activity, making them more effective at clearing out invaders and dead cells. This increased macrophage action supports your immune system's efforts to keep you healthy. It's like giving your body's clean-up crew a boost, ensuring that your internal environment remains pristine and free from harmful substances. Additionally, castor oil's effect on macrophages complements its ability to improve lymphatic drainage, creating a synergistic effect that bolsters your body's natural defenses.

At a molecular level, castor oil works its magic by influencing anti-inflammatory pathways. One of the key mechanisms involved is the inhibition of prostaglandin synthesis. Prostaglandins are lipid compounds that have a role in inflammation and pain signaling. By modulating these compounds, castor oil can reduce inflammation, providing relief from conditions characterized by swelling and discomfort. This anti-inflammatory action is beneficial not only for acute injuries but also for chronic inflammatory conditions. It helps to calm the body's inflammatory response, preventing it from becoming overactive and causing damage to healthy tissues. This soothing effect on inflammation is one of the reasons why castor oil is so widely used in integrative health practices, where it's valued for its ability to complement other treatments and support overall wellness.

Scientific studies have explored the systemic immune benefits of castor oil, revealing its potential to enhance your body's resilience to infections. These studies indicate that regular use of castor oil can lead to an increased production of lymphocytes, the white blood cells responsible for mounting an immune response. Higher lymphocyte levels translate to a more robust immune system, better equipped to fend off viruses, bacteria, and other pathogens. This makes castor oil a valuable ally during times when your immune system might be under particular stress, such as during seasonal changes or periods of increased exposure to germs. By supporting lymphocyte production, castor oil helps maintain a vigilant and responsive immune system, ready to tackle challenges as they arise.

In integrative health practices, castor oil is often used as part of a holistic approach to wellness. Its immune-modulating properties complement other natural therapies, providing a gentle yet effective means of supporting the body's inherent healing abilities. This use of castor oil aligns with a broader understanding of health, where the focus is on nurturing the body's systems to function optimally. Whether you're incorporating castor oil into your routine through topical applications or using it as part of a detox regimen, you're tapping into its rich tapestry of benefits that have been recognized and utilized across cultures for centuries. The science behind castor oil's efficacy in boosting immunity is a testament to nature's wisdom, offering you a simple yet powerful way to support your health in today's complex world.

2.3 Hair Growth Unveiled: Science Behind Castor Oil's Effectiveness

The allure of thick, healthy hair has captivated people for centuries, and castor oil has long been a trusted ally in achieving this. One of the key mechanisms through which castor oil promotes hair growth is by enhancing blood circulation to the scalp. When you massage castor oil into your scalp, it stimulates blood flow, ensuring that hair follicles receive an ample supply of oxygen and nutrients. This nourishment is crucial for hair health, as well-fed follicles can produce stronger and healthier strands. The increased circulation also helps to carry away waste products and toxins that might otherwise impede hair growth. This process is akin to ensuring that a garden is well-watered and free of weeds, allowing the plants to thrive.

In addition to boosting circulation, castor oil is rich in antioxidants, which play a vital role in maintaining hair health. Antioxidants are compounds that help to neutralize free radicals—unstable molecules that can damage cells, including those in your hair. By protecting against free radical damage, castor oil helps to prevent hair thinning and loss, common issues that can arise from oxidative stress. The presence of antioxidants in castor oil acts as a protective shield, safeguarding your hair from environmental damage and keeping it resilient and vibrant. This protection extends to the scalp, where antioxidants help maintain a healthy environment for hair to grow, reducing the likelihood of dandruff and irritation.

The impact of castor oil on the keratin structure of hair is another reason it is cherished for hair care. Keratin is a protein that forms the structural framework of your hair, contributing to its strength and elasticity. Castor oil helps to fortify the keratin in your hair, strengthening the hair shaft and reducing breakage and split ends. This reinforcement is particularly beneficial for those with weak or damaged hair, as it helps to restore vitality and resilience. By applying castor oil regularly, you can enjoy hair that is not only stronger but also more elastic, minimizing the risk of damage from styling and environmental stressors. This strengthening effect is akin to reinforcing a bridge, ensuring that it can withstand the weight and pressure placed upon it.

Clinical studies provide further evidence of castor oil's effectiveness in promoting hair regrowth. Research has shown measurable increases in hair density among individuals using castor oil treatments, offering a tangible testament to its benefits. These studies compare castor oil favorably with other hair growth treatments, highlighting its natural and gentle approach to enhancing hair health. Unlike some chemical treatments that can have harsh side effects, castor oil offers a more holistic solution, working in harmony with your body's natural processes to stimulate hair growth. The evidence from these studies underscores the potential of castor oil to transform hair care routines, offering a natural and effective alternative to conventional treatments.

The effectiveness of castor oil in promoting hair health is a testament to its multifaceted benefits. Whether you are seeking to enhance circulation, protect against damage, or strengthen your hair, castor oil offers a comprehensive solution that addresses multiple aspects of hair health. By incorporating this natural remedy into your hair care routine, you can enjoy the benefits of healthier, stronger, and more resilient hair. The science behind castor oil's effectiveness is a testament to the power of nature, providing a simple yet powerful tool for achieving the hair of your dreams.

2.4 Castor Oil and Digestive Health: A Look at the Science

Imagine the discomfort of a sluggish digestive system. Many find relief from such issues with castor oil, a natural laxative known for its ability to stimulate intestinal peristalsis. Peristalsis is the rhythmic contraction of the muscles in the intestines, which propels waste through the digestive tract. When you consume castor oil, it triggers these contractions, effectively moving stool along and out of the body. This action is not only efficient but also gentle, offering relief without harsh side effects. Additionally, castor oil helps soften stool consistency, making it easier to pass. This is particularly beneficial for those struggling with constipation, where hard stools can cause pain and discomfort. By easing the passage of waste, castor oil supports a more regular and comfortable digestive process.

Beyond its use as a laxative, castor oil has been shown to reduce gut inflammation, making it a valuable tool for managing digestive disorders. Conditions like inflammatory bowel disease (IBD) can cause chronic inflammation in the digestive tract, leading to pain and other symptoms. Castor oil's anti-inflammatory properties help calm this inflammation, providing relief and improving quality of life for those affected. It also reduces intestinal spasms, which are sudden contractions of the intestinal muscles that can cause pain and urgency. By soothing these spasms, castor oil helps maintain a smoother digestive flow, reducing discomfort and allowing the digestive system to function more efficiently. This dual action of reducing inflammation and spasms makes castor oil a multifaceted remedy for digestive health.

The safety profile of castor oil in digestive applications is well-documented, but like any remedy, it requires careful use. Adults are generally advised to take small doses, usually around one to two tablespoons, depending on individual needs and tolerance. It's important to start with a lower dose to assess how your body responds. While castor oil is effective, it can cause side effects such as nausea or abdominal cramping in some individuals. These are usually mild and temporary but should be monitored. Contraindications include certain medical conditions, such as appendicitis or bowel obstruction, where the use of a laxative could exacerbate symptoms. Consulting with a healthcare professional before use, especially if you have underlying health issues, is always recommended.

Emerging research is shedding light on castor oil's interactions with the gut microbiome, the complex community of microorganisms living in your intestines. Recent studies suggest that castor oil may positively impact beneficial gut bacteria, promoting a healthy microbial balance. A balanced microbiome is crucial for digestive health, as it aids in the breakdown of food, supports immune function, and influences overall well-being. By fostering a favorable environment for beneficial bacteria, castor oil may help enhance the health of your gut microbiome. This potential to promote microbial balance is an exciting avenue of research, offering new insights into how castor oil can contribute to digestive health beyond its traditional uses.

As you consider incorporating castor oil into your routine, it's essential to understand its multifaceted role in digestive health. Whether you're seeking relief from constipation, managing a digestive disorder, or looking to support your gut microbiome, castor oil offers a natural and effective option. Its ability to stimulate peristalsis, reduce inflammation, and support microbial balance makes it a versatile tool in promoting digestive wellness. With careful use and an understanding of its benefits, castor oil can be a valuable addition to your health regimen, supporting not only your digestive system but your overall well-being.

As we conclude our exploration of castor oil's scientific foundations, we transition into its practical applications, where historical wisdom and modern science converge to offer tangible benefits in everyday life.

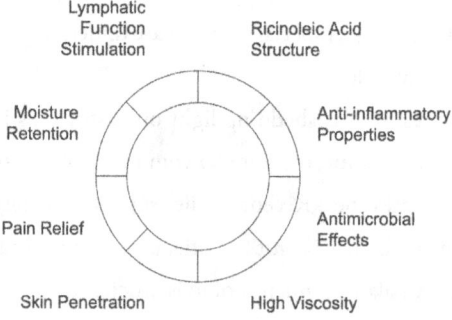

The Multifaceted Benefits of Castor Oil

Chapter 3
Selecting and Storing Authentic Castor Oil

Picture yourself standing in the aisle of a health store, surrounded by shelves lined with countless bottles of castor oil. Each promises purity and effectiveness, but how do you know which one truly delivers? The key lies in understanding the labels. These labels are more than just a list of ingredients; they are a map that guides you to the treasure of pure, authentic castor oil. By learning to decode these labels, you can navigate the market with confidence, ensuring that you choose a product that meets the highest standards of quality and efficacy.

When examining a castor oil label, the first thing to check is the ingredients list. A pure castor oil should stand alone in its ingredient list, free from any additives or fillers. Additives can dilute the oil's potency, while fillers may introduce unwanted chemicals that detract from its natural benefits. Look for labels that proudly display "100% pure castor oil" as this indicates a product that retains the full spectrum of the oil's therapeutic properties. If you see additional ingredients, it's worth reconsidering your choice, as the presence of other substances can compromise the oil's integrity and effectiveness.

Another crucial aspect to consider is the method of extraction, typically noted as "cold-pressed" or "expeller-pressed." Cold-pressed castor oil is extracted without heat, preserving the oil's natural nutrients and active compounds. This method ensures that the oil retains its full range of benefits, from moisturizing properties to anti-inflammatory effects. On the other hand, expeller-pressed oils are produced using heat, which can degrade some of these beneficial compounds. Choosing a cold-pressed oil is akin to selecting the freshest produce at the market; it's about preserving the vitality and potency of the product.

Sourcing information is equally important, as it provides insight into the oil's origins and quality. The origin country can be a telltale sign of an oil's authenticity. Countries like India are renowned for producing high-quality castor oil, thanks to their rich agricultural traditions and expertise in oil extraction. Additionally, look for organic certification, which indicates that the oil is free from pesticides and synthetic fertilizers. Organic certification ensures that the oil is as natural as possible, allowing you to enjoy its benefits without exposure to harmful substances.

The packaging of castor oil is not merely a question of aesthetics; it plays a vital role in maintaining the oil's quality. Dark glass bottles, often amber or cobalt blue, are ideal for storing castor oil. These bottles protect the oil from UV light, which can degrade its quality over time. Just as the sun can fade the colors of a painting, UV exposure can diminish the potency of castor oil, weakening its benefits. A sealed cap is another essential feature, as it prevents contamination and ensures freshness. An improperly sealed bottle can allow air and moisture to enter, compromising the oil's integrity and leading to spoilage.

Understanding expiration dates is crucial for maintaining the effectiveness of your castor oil. The expiration date offers a guideline for the oil's shelf life, indicating when it will begin to lose potency. However, this date is not set in stone. Storage conditions can significantly affect an oil's longevity. For instance, storing the oil in a cool, dark place can extend its shelf life, while exposure to heat and light can accelerate degradation. Think of it as storing a fine wine; the right conditions preserve its quality, allowing you to enjoy its full flavor and aroma even years after purchase.

Interactive Element: Label Decoding Exercise

To put this knowledge into practice, take a moment to examine a bottle of castor oil you have or consider purchasing one for this exercise. Use the following checklist to evaluate the product:

- **Ingredients List**:

Ensure it lists only castor oil with no additives.

- **Extraction Method**:

Check for "cold-pressed" to retain nutrients.

- **Sourcing Information**:

Look for reputable origin countries and organic certification.

- **Packaging**:

Confirm the use of dark glass bottles and sealed caps.

- **Expiration Date**:

Note the date and assess storage conditions.

By completing this exercise, you'll become more adept at selecting authentic castor oil, heightening your confidence as a discerning consumer.

3.1 Certifications and Quality: Ensuring Authenticity

When it comes to selecting castor oil, certifications serve as your beacon of trust, guiding you through a market filled with varied options. One of the most crucial certifications to look for is the USDA Organic label. This certification assures you that the castor oil was produced without synthetic fertilizers, pesticides, or genetically modified organisms. It reflects a commitment to natural farming practices that prioritize environmental health and sustainability. Knowing that a product carries the USDA Organic certification gives you confidence in its purity and quality, ensuring that what you're using is as close to nature as possible. Another important certification is Fair Trade. This label signifies that the farmers and workers involved in producing the castor oil were paid fairly and worked under safe conditions. It represents a dedication to ethical sourcing and social responsibility, ensuring that your purchase supports communities rather than exploiting them.

Third-party testing plays a pivotal role in reinforcing these certifications, offering an additional layer of verification. Independent laboratories conduct purity analysis to confirm that the castor oil meets specific quality standards. They test for contaminants, ensuring that the oil is free from harmful substances like heavy metals and chemical residues. These tests provide an unbiased assessment of the oil's quality, allowing you to make informed decisions. When a brand invests in third-party testing, it demonstrates transparency and accountability, showing that they stand by the quality of their product. This extra step not only confirms the claims made on the label but also builds consumer trust, creating a sense of security in your purchase.

Brand reputation is another significant factor when assessing the quality of castor oil. Established brands with a history of consistent quality often have the trust of the community. They have built their reputation over years, if not decades, and their continued success depends on maintaining high standards. User testimonials and expert endorsements further bolster a brand's credibility. Reading reviews from other consumers can provide insights into the product's real-world performance, while endorsements from experts in the field offer a professional perspective on its efficacy. Together, these elements create a comprehensive picture of a brand's reliability, helping you choose a product that meets your expectations and needs.

Sustainability practices also contribute to the authenticity of castor oil. Ethical sourcing involves sustainable farming practices that protect the environment and support biodiversity. By choosing oils produced through sustainable methods, you contribute to efforts that preserve the planet's resources for future generations. Community support initiatives further enhance a brand's authenticity. Companies that invest in the communities where their products are sourced demonstrate a commitment to social responsibility. These initiatives might include educational programs, health services, or infrastructure development, providing tangible benefits to local populations. Supporting brands that engage in these practices ensures that your purchase is part of a larger positive impact, extending the benefits of your choice beyond personal health to global well-being.

3.2 Storage Solutions: Preserving Potency and Freshness

Imagine you've just brought home a bottle of high-quality castor oil, full of potential to enhance your health and beauty routines. To maintain its potency and effectiveness, proper storage is key. Castor oil, like many natural oils, is sensitive to environmental factors that can degrade its quality over time. Temperature control is one of the most crucial elements to consider. Heat exposure can accelerate the breakdown of its beneficial compounds, diminishing its therapeutic properties. It's best to store your castor oil in a cool, stable environment, away from heat sources such as radiators or direct sunlight. The pantry or a cupboard can be ideal spots, as long as they maintain a consistent temperature. Extreme temperature fluctuations, like those experienced in an unregulated garage or attic, can wreak havoc on your oil's quality.

The impact of temperature fluctuations on castor oil should not be underestimated. When oil is repeatedly exposed to varying temperatures, it can lead to the separation of components, affecting its texture and efficacy. Refrigeration, although seemingly a good idea, can cause the oil to thicken excessively, making it difficult to use. Freezing is even more detrimental, as it can lead to permanent changes in texture and possibly spoil the oil. Therefore, maintaining a stable, moderate temperature is far more beneficial than storing it in extreme cold. If you find your storage space tends to get warm, consider adding a small fan or placing the oil in a cooler part of your home to prevent any adverse effects of heat.

Choosing the right container for your castor oil is another vital consideration. Airtight glass containers are the best choice, as they prevent air from entering and oxidizing the oil. Oxidation can lead to rancidity, altering the oil's smell and effectiveness. Glass is inert, meaning it doesn't interact with the oil, preserving its purity and integrity. Avoid plastic containers, as they can leach chemicals into the oil, especially when exposed to heat, compromising its quality. Furthermore, plastic is slightly permeable, allowing air and moisture to seep in over time. This gradual exposure can lead to degradation, affecting both the scent and performance of the oil. When transferring oil from its original packaging, use a clean, dry glass bottle to ensure optimal preservation.

Extending the shelf life of your castor oil involves a few practical steps. Adding natural preservatives like vitamin E can help maintain its freshness. Vitamin E acts as an antioxidant, delaying the oxidation process and keeping the oil stable for a longer period. Regularly checking your oil for signs of rancidity is also important. A telltale sign of spoilage is a sour or off-putting smell. If the oil's aroma has shifted from its natural, mild scent to something unpleasant, it might be time to replace it. Additionally, observe the oil's color and consistency. Pure castor oil should remain clear and viscous. Cloudiness or separation may indicate that the oil has started to degrade. By staying vigilant and taking these preventive measures, you can ensure that your castor oil remains effective and ready for use whenever you need it.

Creating a routine for checking the quality of your castor oil is helpful. Mark your calendar to inspect it every few months, noting any changes in appearance or scent. This proactive approach allows you to catch any issues early, ensuring that your oil stays in top condition. You might also find it useful to label your bottles with the date of purchase. This helps track how long the oil has been stored and guides you in using it before it reaches the end of its shelf life. By incorporating these small habits into your routine, you cultivate a mindful approach to storage, enhancing your experience with this versatile oil. Taking these steps not only preserves the oil's quality but also maximizes its benefits, allowing you to enjoy its full potential.

3.3 Recognizing Adulterated Products: Red Flags to Watch For

In the bustling market of natural oils, it can be a challenge to identify which products are truly pure and which have been compromised. Adulteration is a common issue, where cheaper substances are mixed with oils to cut costs, often at the expense of quality and safety. Identifying these adulterated products requires a keen eye and a bit of know-how. One of the first signs to look for is an unusual scent. Pure castor oil typically has a mild, nutty aroma that is not overpowering. If you detect a strong, chemical-like smell or an off-putting odor, it could indicate the presence of additives or impurities that shouldn't be there.

Color is another clue. Authentic castor oil is usually pale yellow or colorless. If the oil appears dark yellow, brown, or cloudy, it may have been contaminated. Cloudiness, in particular, suggests the presence of unwanted particles or emulsifiers, which can alter the oil's natural properties. Similarly, if you notice any separation of layers or sediment at the bottom of the bottle, this could be a red flag. Pure castor oil should have a consistent texture and appearance throughout. These visual cues are often the first indications that an oil is not what it claims to be.

At home, you can conduct a few simple tests to further verify the purity of your castor oil. One such method is the solubility test. Pure castor oil does not dissolve in alcohol, so when mixed, it should separate rather than blend smoothly. This test can help you determine whether the oil has been mixed with other substances that might dissolve more readily. Consistency checks are also valuable. Genuine castor oil is thick and viscous, with a slightly sticky feel. If your oil feels thin or watery, it may have been diluted with a lighter, less expensive oil. These tests offer a practical, hands-on way to assess the quality of your oil without specialized equipment.

Using adulterated castor oil can pose several risks. Aside from diminishing the oil's therapeutic benefits, impurities can lead to skin irritation or allergic reactions. The skin, being the body's largest organ and first line of defense, can react negatively to foreign substances. This is particularly concerning for individuals with sensitive skin or existing conditions like eczema or psoriasis. Additionally, the efficacy of the oil in promoting hair growth, soothing inflammation, or moisturizing skin is greatly reduced if it is not pure. When you apply adulterated oil, you may not receive the full spectrum of benefits you expect or need, leading to disappointment and potential health issues.

To avoid these risks, it's crucial to exercise vigilance when purchasing castor oil.

- Opt for trusted retailers known for their commitment to quality and transparency. These businesses often provide detailed information about their sourcing and production processes, offering reassurance about the product's purity.

- Be wary of prices that seem too good to be true. While everyone loves a bargain, an exceptionally low price may indicate that the product has been compromised in some way. True quality comes at a cost, reflecting the care and integrity involved in producing a pure, effective oil.

In your journey of selecting the right castor oil, it's beneficial to cultivate a sense of discernment. By paying attention to the signs of adulteration and conducting your own tests, you empower yourself to make informed choices. This vigilance not only protects you from subpar products but also enhances your experience with castor oil, ensuring that you reap all the benefits this natural wonder has to offer.

In conclusion, navigating the world of castor oil requires a blend of knowledge and attentiveness. Recognizing signs of adulteration, understanding the risks of impure products, and practicing smart purchasing habits all contribute to a more rewarding and safe use of castor oil. As we move forward, we'll explore the diverse applications and benefits of this remarkable oil, building on the foundation of authenticity and quality we've established.

Castor Oil Storage Cycle

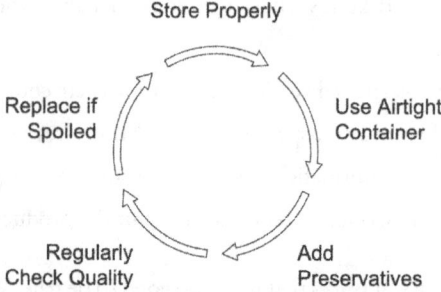

Chapter 4
Practical Applications for Health and Wellness

Picture a humble bottle of castor oil sitting unassumingly in your bathroom cabinet. Its potential might surprise you, as this age-old remedy holds the power of a natural pharmacy. The ancient wisdom surrounding castor oil is matched by modern science, unveiling a myriad of health benefits. This thick, golden liquid is more than a household staple—it's a versatile tool for your well-being. As you explore its uses, you'll find that castor oil can address a range of health concerns, from inflammation to detoxification, offering a natural alternative to synthetic products. Let's delve into how castor oil can become a cornerstone of your health and wellness routine.

Castor oil's anti-inflammatory and antimicrobial effects are among its most celebrated properties, making it a valuable ally in soothing irritated skin and combating infections. As we have discussed, the oil's primary component, ricinoleic acid, is a potent anti-inflammatory agent that can reduce swelling and redness when applied topically. This makes it particularly effective for treating conditions like acne, psoriasis, and eczema, where inflammation is a common concern. Moreover, its antimicrobial properties help prevent infection by inhibiting the growth of bacteria and fungi. This dual action makes castor oil an excellent choice for maintaining healthy skin and preventing common dermatological issues. By incorporating castor oil into your skincare regimen, you can harness its natural healing power to promote a clearer, healthier complexion.

The oil's antioxidant properties contribute significantly to cellular health, protecting your body from the damaging effects of free radicals. These unstable molecules can cause oxidative stress, leading to cell damage and contributing to the aging process. Castor oil is rich in antioxidants, which neutralize free radicals and support cellular repair and regeneration. This not only helps maintain youthful skin but also supports overall health by protecting vital organs and tissues from oxidative damage. By using castor oil regularly, you can bolster your body's defenses against the wear and tear of daily life, promoting longevity and vitality. Its role as an antioxidant makes castor oil a valuable addition to any health-conscious individual's routine.

Beyond skincare, castor oil impacts hormone balance, an often-overlooked aspect of health. Hormonal imbalances can manifest in various ways, from mood swings to weight fluctuations, affecting both men and women. Castor oil supports hormonal equilibrium by enhancing the function of the endocrine system, which regulates hormone production and release. This can be particularly beneficial for women experiencing menstrual irregularities or menopause symptoms, as it helps stabilize hormone levels and alleviate associated discomforts. Regular use of castor oil, whether through topical application or as part of a holistic routine, can aid in maintaining hormonal balance, contributing to a sense of overall well-being and stability.

The oil's role in detoxification and lymphatic health further underscores its versatility as a natural remedy. The lymphatic system, a crucial component of the body's immune defense, relies on movement and drainage to remove toxins and waste products. Castor oil enhances lymphatic circulation, facilitating the elimination of these substances and supporting detoxification processes. This can lead to improved energy levels, reduced bloating, and better overall health. By applying castor oil to areas like the abdomen or lymph nodes, you can stimulate lymphatic flow and encourage your body's natural cleansing mechanisms. This practice not only aids in detoxification but also boosts immune function, helping you stay resilient and healthy.

Reflection Section: Exploring Your Needs

Consider your current health routine. Are there areas where you feel castor oil could offer support, such as skincare, hormone balance, or detoxification? Take a moment to reflect on how incorporating castor oil could enhance your well-being. Imagine the changes you would like to see and how this natural remedy might assist in achieving them. Write down your thoughts and goals to keep track of your journey with castor oil.

4.1 Boosting Immunity: Daily Rituals with Castor Oil

Incorporating castor oil into your daily routine can significantly benefit your immune system. This natural oil serves as a gentle yet powerful immune-boosting agent. One effective practice is the morning oil-pulling ritual. This involves swishing a tablespoon of castor oil in your mouth for about 15 minutes, then spitting it out. This simple act not only promotes oral health by reducing bacteria but also supports overall immune function. Starting your day with this ritual can set a tone of mindfulness and self-care, anchoring you in a routine that enhances your health from within.

Another beneficial practice is a castor oil foot massage, which improves circulation and supports immune health. By massaging your feet with castor oil, you stimulate blood flow, providing a soothing end to your day while also promoting better circulation. This practice can lead to improved oxygen delivery and nutrient absorption throughout your body, supporting the immune system in its vital role of defending against pathogens. It's a straightforward way to nurture your body, offering relaxation and immune support in one calming ritual.

Applying castor oil on lymph nodes is another daily practice to consider. The lymphatic system plays a crucial role in immune function, and castor oil can enhance lymphatic flow, aiding in the removal of toxins. Gently massaging castor oil over areas like the neck, armpits, or groin can help keep your lymphatic system functioning optimally. Complementing this, preparing a soothing castor oil tea can provide internal support. By combining castor oil with warm water and a touch of honey, you create a comforting beverage that hydrates and nourishes, offering a gentle boost to your immune system.

As seasons change, so do the challenges your immune system faces. During colder months, adjusting your use of castor oil can provide added support. For instance, applying a warming layer of castor oil on your chest can offer comfort and protection against winter's chill. Pairing castor oil with herbal teas like echinacea can further enhance its immune-boosting effects. The combination of these natural remedies can help fortify your immune defenses, keeping you resilient in the face of seasonal shifts.

The synergy of castor oil with other immune-boosting practices offers a holistic approach to health. Pairing it with vitamin C-rich foods can amplify its benefits, as vitamin C is renowned for its role in supporting immune function. Additionally, incorporating mindfulness and stress reduction techniques, such as meditation or deep breathing exercises, can further enhance the effects of castor oil. Stress can weaken your immune system, so by combining these practices, you create a comprehensive routine that addresses both physical and mental well-being.

In exploring these practices, consider how you can seamlessly integrate them into your daily life. Whether it's through a morning ritual, an evening massage, or simple dietary adjustments, castor oil offers numerous ways to support your immune health. These practices not only boost your immune system but also foster a deeper connection to your body's needs, promoting a balanced and resilient state of health. Embracing these rituals can transform your daily routine, making wellness an intrinsic part of your lifestyle.

4.2 Natural Pain Relief: Castor Oil for Muscle and Joint Comfort

Imagine coming home after a long day, your muscles aching from exertion. The thought of relief, soothing and natural, might lead you to consider the analgesic properties of castor oil. This oil, with its rich, viscous consistency, offers comfort to tired and sore muscles. When combined with essential oils like lavender, it transforms into a calming balm, perfect for massage. Lavender, known for its relaxing scent and anti-inflammatory properties, complements castor oil beautifully. Together, they create a blend that not only eases tension but also calms the mind. As you massage this blend into your muscles, feel the relief washing over you, the oil penetrating deep to relax and rejuvenate.

To make a muscle-relief balm, start with a base of castor oil. Add a few drops of lavender essential oil and mix well. You might also include eucalyptus or peppermint oil for an invigorating touch. These oils enhance circulation and provide a cooling sensation that further eases discomfort. For a joint-relief soak, dissolve Epsom salts in a warm bath and add a generous splash of your castor oil blend. Soak for twenty minutes, allowing the warmth to open your pores and the oils to penetrate deeply. This combination soothes inflammation and relaxes the body, leaving you refreshed and pain-free.

Applying castor oil as a warm compress enhances its pain-relieving effects. Heat increases blood flow to affected areas, helping the oil penetrate deeper into tissues. Simply soak a cloth in castor oil, apply it to the sore area, and cover with a heating pad. The warmth not only soothes aching muscles but also amplifies the oil's therapeutic properties, providing a comforting, effective relief. Regular use can significantly reduce muscle stiffness and joint pain, making it a valuable addition to any pain management routine.

Real-life testimonials highlight the effectiveness of castor oil in pain relief. Athletes, who often push their bodies to the limit, find comfort in its soothing properties. One marathon runner shared how a daily castor oil massage helped alleviate post-run soreness, allowing for quicker recovery and better performance. Similarly, individuals with arthritis praise its ability to ease chronic joint pain. One arthritis patient recounted their experience, noting how castor oil compresses provided a natural alternative to over-the-counter pain medications. These stories underscore the potential of castor oil as a natural remedy, offering relief without the side effects of traditional painkillers.

4.3 Enhancing Digestion: Recipes and Techniques

Imagine sitting down for a meal and knowing that you're doing more than just satisfying hunger—you're nurturing your digestive system. Castor oil, with its gentle laxative effects, can be your ally in promoting digestive health. It works by stimulating the intestinal muscles, encouraging regular bowel movements, and providing relief from occasional constipation. This natural approach avoids the harshness of some chemical laxatives, allowing your body to function smoothly. Moreover, castor oil supports liver function by improving bile flow, which is essential for digesting fats and detoxifying the body. This dual action helps maintain a balanced digestive system and contributes to overall well-being.

For those interested in incorporating castor oil into their daily routine, consider starting your morning with a digestive tonic. Combine a small amount of castor oil with warm water and lemon juice. This simple concoction can kickstart your digestive system, preparing it for the day ahead. In the evening, a soothing elixir can help wind down your digestive process. Mix castor oil with herbal tea, such as chamomile or peppermint, to create a calming beverage that aids digestion while promoting relaxation. These recipes are easy to prepare and integrate into your day, offering subtle support to your digestive health.

Incorporating castor oil into meals can be an effective way to enjoy its benefits without altering your diet drastically. Try drizzling a small amount over salads or soups. Its subtle nutty flavor can enhance the dish while supporting digestion. Another option is blending it into smoothies. A teaspoon of castor oil can add a smooth texture and nutritional boost. These methods allow you to enjoy the oil's benefits seamlessly, without needing to change your culinary habits significantly. It's about enhancing what you already love to eat with a touch of wellness.

Safety and dosage considerations are important when using castor oil internally. For adults, a recommended dose typically ranges from one to two teaspoons, but it's wise to start small and observe how your body responds. Those with specific health conditions, such as pregnant women or individuals with gastrointestinal disorders, should consult a healthcare professional before use. Castor oil's potency requires respect, and understanding your body's needs ensures a positive experience. Always remember that moderation is key, and listening to your body's signals can guide you in finding the perfect balance.

Exploring castor oil's role in digestion opens up a world of natural health solutions. Its ability to support regularity and liver function makes it a valuable tool in maintaining digestive health. The simple act of incorporating it into your diet can lead to noticeable improvements in how you feel, both physically and mentally. By choosing to integrate castor oil into your routine, you're embracing a holistic approach to wellness, one that values balance and natural remedies. This journey of exploration can reveal new ways to care for yourself, fostering a deeper connection with your body's needs and rhythms.

4.4 Castor Oil Packs: A Step-by-Step Guide for Internal Healing

The concept of castor oil packs might seem simple at first glance, yet their benefits run deep. These packs are a gentle way to promote internal healing, offering a natural method for improving well-being. Castor oil packs are renowned for their ability to aid liver detoxification, helping the body eliminate toxins more efficiently. The liver, our body's primary detox organ, often bears the burden of modern life. By applying a castor oil pack to the abdomen, you can support liver function, enhancing its ability to cleanse the bloodstream. This practice can lead to increased energy levels, clearer skin, and improved digestion.

Beyond detoxification, castor oil packs are also useful for reducing menstrual cramps. Many women experience discomfort during their menstrual cycle, and the soothing warmth of a castor oil pack can provide much-needed relief. Applied to the lower abdomen, the pack helps relax uterine muscles, reducing cramping and promoting relaxation. This natural approach offers a gentle alternative to over-the-counter pain medications, allowing you to manage menstrual discomfort with a simple, at-home remedy.

Creating a castor oil pack is straightforward. You'll need a piece of unbleached wool or cotton flannel, a bottle of high-quality castor oil, a plastic sheet, and a heating pad. Start by cutting the fabric into several layers, then saturate them with castor oil. Place the soaked fabric on a plastic sheet to prevent staining, then apply it to the desired area of your body. Cover it with the plastic sheet and add a heating pad on top. The heat will help the oil penetrate the skin, enhancing its therapeutic effects. Leave the pack in place for at least 45 minutes to an hour, allowing the oil to work its magic.

The applications of castor oil packs are diverse. When placed on the abdomen, they can improve digestive health by encouraging bowel movements and reducing bloating. For those with arthritis, applying a pack to affected joints can provide relief by reducing inflammation and improving circulation. The warmth and pressure of the pack help relax tense muscles and joints, offering a soothing experience. This versatility makes castor oil packs a valuable tool for addressing various health concerns, from digestive issues to joint pain.

Holistic health practitioners have long praised the benefits of castor oil packs. Many naturopaths recommend them for their ability to stimulate the body's natural healing processes. According to holistic coach Sarah Lane, "Castor oil packs are a gentle and effective way to support the body's detox pathways, promoting overall wellness." These endorsements from experts in natural health highlight the packs' efficacy, providing reassurance to those looking to incorporate them into their wellness routine.

For those seeking a natural approach to health, castor oil packs offer a simple yet powerful solution. Whether you're using them for detoxification, menstrual relief, or joint pain, these packs provide a versatile method for supporting your body's needs. Their ease of use and broad applications make them an accessible option for anyone interested in exploring the benefits of natural healing. As you incorporate castor oil packs into your routine, you'll discover the profound impact they can have on your health and well-being.

4.5 Detoxifying the Body: Integrating Castor Oil into Cleansing Practices

In the quest for holistic health, detoxification has become a pillar of wellness. Castor oil stands out as a powerful ally in this process, offering a natural means to support the body's cleansing efforts.

Stimulating the Lymphatic System

One of its most remarkable roles is in aiding lymphatic drainage, crucial for removing toxins and waste from the body. The lymphatic system, often called the body's drainage network, relies on movement and flow to function effectively. Applying castor oil to areas like the neck and armpits can stimulate this system, promoting the removal of cellular waste and enhancing overall health. This practice not only cleanses but revitalizes, leaving you feeling lighter and more energized.

Detox Castor Oil Bath

Detoxifying the skin is another area where castor oil excels. A detoxifying castor oil bath can be a restorative ritual, drawing impurities out and leaving the skin refreshed. To create this bath, mix a few tablespoons of castor oil with Epsom salts and add to warm water. The combination works wonders, opening pores and promoting the release of toxins. As you soak, the oil's emollient properties soothe and hydrate, transforming your bath into a spa-like experience. This practice can be especially beneficial after a long day, helping to unwind and cleanse both body and mind.

Dry brushing

Pairing castor oil with other detox methods enhances its effects, creating a comprehensive cleansing routine. Dry brushing is a popular technique that, when used with castor oil, can amplify results. Before showering, gently brush your skin with a natural bristle brush, then apply castor oil to the skin. This combination exfoliates and encourages lymphatic flow, making detoxification more effective. Similarly, incorporating detoxifying herbs like dandelion root can support liver function and improve digestion. A herbal tea blended with a hint of castor oil offers a dual-action approach, cleansing internally while nourishing from within.

As with any detox practice, it's important to be aware of potential detox symptoms. These can include fatigue, headaches, or minor skin irritations as the body adjusts and releases toxins. Staying hydrated is crucial during this time, as water assists in flushing out impurities. Rest is equally important, allowing the body to recover and adapt. If symptoms persist, consider reducing the frequency or intensity of your detox routine and gradually build up as your body acclimates. Listening to your body's signals ensures a safe and effective detox experience, optimizing the benefits of castor oil.

Detoxifying with castor oil is as much about creating a mindful practice as it is about physical cleansing. It's an opportunity to slow down, connect with your body, and embrace a natural approach to health. The versatility of castor oil allows it to fit seamlessly into various detox routines, offering support tailored to individual needs. Whether you're soaking in a detox bath or enhancing your skincare with castor oil, you're engaging in a ritual that nurtures both body and spirit. This holistic perspective is key to understanding the depth of benefits castor oil can provide, paving the way for a healthier, more balanced life.

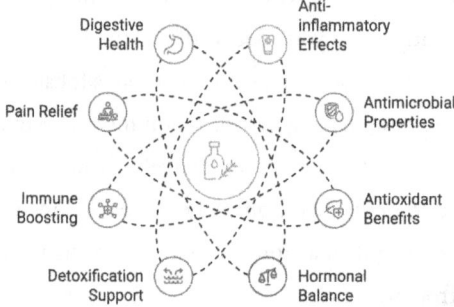

Chapter 5
Beauty and Personal Care with Castor Oil

Imagine holding a bottle of castor oil and considering its potential to transform your skincare routine. This ancient oil, once used by our ancestors for its healing properties, has made its way into modern beauty regimens due to its versatility and effectiveness. Whether you're looking to hydrate your skin, balance oil production, or soothe sensitivity, castor oil can be a valuable ally. Its emollient properties help maintain skin hydration and softness, making it a staple for those seeking radiant, healthy skin. Let's explore how this remarkable oil can enrich your beauty rituals and support a natural approach to skincare.

5.1 DIY Skincare: Radiant Skin with Castor Oil

Castor oil is a versatile skincare ingredient known for its ability to lock in moisture and create a protective barrier on the skin. Its thick consistency makes it particularly effective for dry skin, where it acts as an occlusive moisturizer, preventing water loss and keeping the skin supple. By mixing castor oil with rosehip oil, you can create a hydrating face serum. Rosehip oil, rich in vitamins A and C, complements castor oil by promoting skin regeneration and reducing the appearance of scars and fine lines. This combination offers a nourishing treatment that can be applied nightly, leaving your skin feeling rejuvenated and glowing by morning.

Castor oil's benefits extend to various skin types, including oily and combination skin. Its low comedogenic score means it's unlikely to clog pores, making it suitable even for those prone to acne. For combination skin, a balancing facial oil can be formulated by blending castor oil with a lighter carrier oil, such as jojoba or grapeseed. This blend helps regulate oil production while providing hydration where needed. For sensitive skin, a soothing mask can be crafted using castor oil and oatmeal. Oatmeal's calming properties, combined with castor oil's moisturizing effects, create a mask that soothes irritation and redness, offering relief to delicate skin.

Creating your own skincare products at home allows you to tailor them to your specific needs. A rejuvenating overnight cream can be made by mixing castor oil with shea butter and a few drops of lavender essential oil. The shea butter adds richness and nourishment, while lavender provides calming effects that promote restful sleep. For exfoliation, a castor sugar scrub is a simple yet effective recipe. Combine castor oil with fine sugar and a touch of honey to create a scrub that gently removes dead skin cells, leaving your skin smooth and polished. These DIY recipes not only enhance your skincare routine but also offer a sense of accomplishment and personalization.

Customizing your skincare routine with castor oil is a rewarding experience. By adjusting the consistency with different carrier oils, you can fine-tune the texture to suit your preferences. For a lighter feel, blend castor oil with sunflower or hemp oil. Adding essential oils like chamomile or tea tree can target specific concerns, such as inflammation or breakouts. This flexibility allows you to create products that cater to your unique skin needs while enjoying the therapeutic benefits of natural ingredients. As you experiment with different formulations, you'll discover new ways to care for your skin, making castor oil an integral part of your beauty regimen.

Reflection Section: Personalizing Your Skincare Routine

Take a moment to reflect on your current skincare needs. Are there specific concerns you'd like to address, such as dryness, sensitivity, or oiliness? Consider how castor oil can be incorporated into your routine to support these needs. Jot down a few ideas for DIY recipes you might try, and think about the essential oils or additional ingredients that could enhance your formulations. This exercise encourages you to take an active role in your skincare journey, empowering you to create products that are perfectly suited to your skin's unique requirements.

5.2 Luscious Locks: Hair Treatment Recipes

Imagine running your fingers through your hair, feeling its strength and vitality. This can be your reality with the help of castor oil. Known for its ability to promote hair growth, strength, and shine, castor oil is a celebrated ingredient in hair care. It nourishes the scalp and provides essential nutrients to hair follicles, encouraging new growth and preventing hair loss. Compared to other popular oils like coconut and argan, castor oil's unique composition of fatty acids makes it a superior choice for those seeking to enhance hair health. While coconut oil is known for its deep conditioning properties and argan oil for its light touch and shine, castor oil offers a thick, rich treatment that penetrates deeply, providing a robust solution for various hair concerns.

For those looking to embrace the benefits of castor oil, a deep-conditioning mask is a great place to start. This mask combines three tablespoons of castor oil with one tablespoon of avocado oil and a few drops of lavender essential oil. Avocado oil is rich in vitamin

E and healthy fats, which complement castor oil's properties, while lavender adds a soothing fragrance and promotes relaxation. Apply this mixture to clean, dry hair, focusing on the ends and any areas of dryness. Leave it on for 20 to 30 minutes, allowing the oils to penetrate and hydrate each strand deeply. Rinse thoroughly with warm water and a gentle shampoo, and enjoy the softness and luster that remain.

A scalp-stimulating tonic can also be a valuable addition to your hair care routine. Mix two tablespoons of castor oil with two tablespoons of jojoba oil and a few drops of rosemary essential oil. This combination not only nourishes the scalp but also stimulates blood flow, promoting hair growth. Jojoba oil is known for its similarity to the natural oils produced by the scalp, making it an ideal carrier for castor oil. Rosemary oil, on the other hand, is renowned for its ability to improve circulation and stimulate hair follicles. To apply, massage the tonic into your scalp using gentle, circular motions. This technique not only ensures optimal absorption but also boosts circulation, delivering nutrients directly to the hair roots.

Integrating castor oil into your regular hair care routine is simple and effective. For enhanced penetration, try using a warm towel wrap after applying your chosen treatment. The heat opens up the hair cuticles, allowing the oil to penetrate more deeply and work its magic from within. Simply soak a towel in hot water, wring it out, and wrap it around your head. This spa-like experience enhances the benefits of castor oil, leaving your hair feeling incredibly soft and manageable. For best results, use castor oil treatments once or twice a week, adjusting the frequency based on your hair type and needs. Those with dry or damaged hair may benefit from more frequent applications, while those with oily hair might prefer a more spaced-out approach.

Consider combining castor oil with your favorite leave-in conditioner for daily use. This combination provides ongoing nourishment and protection, keeping your hair healthy and strong between treatments. By adding a few drops of castor oil to your conditioner, you can create a custom blend that addresses your specific hair concerns. This simple tweak to your routine ensures that your hair receives the benefits of castor oil consistently, promoting long-term health and vitality. Whether you're seeking to combat dryness, boost shine, or encourage growth, castor oil can be a transformative addition to your hair care arsenal.

5.3 Castor Oil in Anti-Aging Regimens: Natural Youthfulness

Picture a smooth, youthful complexion that seems to defy the passage of time. Castor oil holds the secret to such timeless beauty thanks to its unique anti-aging properties. Its ability to combat the appearance of wrinkles and fine lines is attributed to its high content of antioxidants. These molecules are crucial in neutralizing free radicals, which are unstable atoms that can damage cells, leading to premature aging. By integrating castor oil into your skincare routine, you provide your skin with a powerful shield against these damaging forces. This protection not only slows down the aging process but also enhances the skin's natural glow, making it appear more vibrant and youthful.

Creating your own anti-aging skincare products at home can be both rewarding and effective. Consider crafting an anti-aging night serum using castor oil and vitamin E. Vitamin E is a potent antioxidant that supports skin repair and regeneration while providing additional moisturization. To make this serum, combine a tablespoon of castor oil with a few drops of vitamin E oil. Apply it to your face before bed, allowing it to work overnight. This simple yet powerful blend can help replenish your skin, reducing the appearance of fine lines and maintaining a youthful look. For the delicate area around your eyes, a firming eye cream with caffeine extract can be incredibly beneficial.

Caffeine helps tighten the skin and reduce puffiness, making it an ideal partner for castor oil's moisturizing effects. By gently applying this cream each morning, you can awaken the eye area, reducing signs of fatigue and enhancing your overall appearance.

One of the most remarkable benefits of castor oil is its ability to improve skin elasticity. As we age, our skin tends to lose its firmness, leading to sagging and the formation of wrinkles. Castor oil aids in enhancing collagen production, a protein that provides structure and strength to the skin. By promoting collagen synthesis, castor oil helps maintain the skin's elasticity, resulting in a firmer, more youthful appearance. Additionally, its ability to smooth uneven skin texture makes it a valuable tool in achieving a polished and refined look. Whether you're dealing with rough patches or uneven skin tone, castor oil can help create a smoother, more even complexion.

The effectiveness of castor oil in anti-aging regimens is supported by both experts and enthusiasts. Dermatologists often highlight its potential to hydrate and protect the skin, noting its use as a natural alternative to harsh chemical treatments. Many skincare enthusiasts share success stories of how castor oil has transformed their routines, citing improvements in skin texture and a reduction in visible signs of aging. One user expressed delight at how castor oil had become a staple in her skincare arsenal, helping her maintain a youthful glow without resorting to expensive products. These testimonials underscore the real-world impact of castor oil, offering reassurance to those considering it for their own anti-aging needs.

5.4 Nail and Cuticle Care: Strengthening with Castor Oil

Imagine your nails, healthy and strong, free from brittleness and breakage. Castor oil can help you achieve this. Its nourishing properties make it an excellent choice for promoting nail health and preventing brittleness. Rich in fatty acids, castor oil penetrates deeply, hydrating the nail bed and surrounding skin. This hydration is crucial for maintaining flexibility and strength, reducing the risk of cracks and splits. Compared to other popular nail oils like jojoba and almond, castor oil stands out for its thicker consistency and ability to provide long-lasting moisture. While jojoba oil is lightweight and quickly absorbed, and almond oil offers a vitamin-rich boost, castor oil's emollient properties ensure it stays where it's needed, offering prolonged nourishment and protection.

Creating your own nail and cuticle care treatments at home is both simple and rewarding.

- A strengthening nail soak can be made by mixing equal parts of castor oil and olive oil in a small bowl.

- Add a few drops of lemon juice for its natural bleaching and antibacterial properties.

- Soak your nails for 10 to 15 minutes, allowing the oils to penetrate and nourish.

- This soak not only strengthens the nails but also promotes a healthier appearance.

- For a hydrating cuticle balm, blend castor oil with shea butter and a few drops of vitamin E oil.

- Heat the mixture gently until combined, then pour it into a small container.

- Once cooled, apply the balm to your cuticles daily, massaging it in to promote absorption and hydration. This balm helps keep cuticles soft and supple, preventing hangnails and promoting overall nail health.

Applying castor oil to your nails is most effective when done at night. Before bed, massage a generous amount of castor oil into your nails and cuticles. To maximize absorption and benefits, slip on a pair of cotton gloves. The warmth from the gloves helps the oil penetrate deeply, providing intensive nourishment while you sleep. This nighttime treatment is an easy way to incorporate castor oil into your routine, ensuring your nails receive the care they deserve without taking time out of your busy day.

Enhancing your nail care routine with regular maintenance practices can amplify the benefits of castor oil. Consider incorporating biotin supplements into your diet, as they are known to support nail strength and growth. Biotin, a B-vitamin, plays a vital role in producing keratin, the protein that forms the structure of nails. By combining internal support with external care, you create a comprehensive approach to nail health. Regular filing and trimming techniques are also important. Use a fine-grit file to shape your nails, smoothing any rough edges that could snag or tear. Trim your nails regularly to maintain a manageable length, reducing the likelihood of breakage. By adopting these practices alongside castor oil treatments, you ensure your nails remain strong, healthy, and beautiful.

Incorporating these tips into your routine allows you to enjoy the full benefits of castor oil for nail and cuticle care. Whether you're creating a relaxing soak, applying a nourishing balm, or enhancing your routine with supplements, castor oil offers a natural solution for maintaining nail health. Its versatility and effectiveness make it an invaluable addition to your beauty regimen, supporting the vitality and strength of your nails with every use.

5.5 Natural Makeup Remover: A Gentle Alternative

Imagine coming home after a long day, your face still adorned with the makeup that has shielded you from the world. The desire for a gentle, effective way to remove it is universal. Castor oil steps in as a natural alternative, offering a way to dissolve makeup effortlessly while nourishing your skin. Its thick consistency makes it particularly effective at breaking down stubborn products, such as waterproof mascara and long-wear lipstick. The oil's gentle nature ensures compatibility with even the most sensitive skin types, providing a soothing cleanse without irritation. Unlike commercial removers, which often contain harsh chemicals and preservatives, castor oil offers a pure, skin-friendly option that leaves your face feeling refreshed and cared for.

To harness these benefits, you can create a simple DIY makeup remover using castor oil and rose water. The combination not only cleanses but also hydrates and tones, thanks to rose water's natural astringent properties. A dual-phase makeup remover combines these two ingredients to create a powerful yet gentle formula.

- Start by pouring one part castor oil and one part rose water into a small bottle.

- Shake well before each use to blend the layers. This mixture effectively lifts away makeup while imparting a touch of luxury to your routine. The soothing scent of rose water adds an element of relaxation, turning makeup removal into a pampering ritual.

When using castor oil as a makeup remover, application techniques can enhance its effectiveness. Begin by saturating a cotton pad with the dual-phase mixture. Gently press the pad onto your skin, allowing the oil to break down the makeup. This technique is particularly effective for eye makeup, where gentle pressure helps dissolve product without tugging on the delicate skin. After the oil has done its work, rinse your face with warm water, ensuring you wash away any residue. This step is crucial to prevent any leftover oil from clogging pores. Follow with your regular cleanser for a double-cleansing routine that leaves your skin impeccably clean and balanced.

The advantages of using natural alternatives like castor oil over commercial makeup removers are compelling. By avoiding harsh chemicals and preservatives, you reduce the risk of skin irritation and allergic reactions. Many commercial products rely on synthetic ingredients that can strip the skin of its natural oils, leading to dryness and imbalance. Castor oil, on the other hand, preserves the skin's moisture barrier, maintaining hydration while cleansing. Additionally, choosing castor oil as your makeup remover contributes to environmental sustainability. By creating your own products, you reduce packaging waste and reliance on single-use items. This conscious choice aligns with a holistic approach to beauty, where caring for yourself goes hand in hand with caring for the planet.

As you integrate castor oil into your beauty routine, you'll discover a newfound appreciation for the simplicity and efficacy of natural ingredients. This approach not only enhances your skin health but also fosters a deeper connection to the products you use daily. With each application, you're making a choice that supports both personal well-being and environmental responsibility. In this way, castor oil transcends its role as a mere beauty product, becoming a symbol of mindful living. The benefits of castor oil extend beyond cleansing, inviting you to explore its potential as a versatile tool in your beauty arsenal. From skincare to hair care, and now makeup removal, castor oil proves itself time and again as a gentle, effective, and sustainable choice for beauty enthusiasts everywhere. Embrace its potential and experience the transformation it offers, both for your skin and your lifestyle.

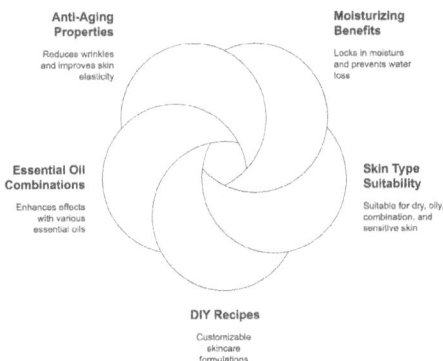

Castor Oil in Skincare

A note from Barbara

As the author of *The Hidden Power of Castor Oil: Nature's Ultimate Elixir Revealed*, I feel honoured to guide you through the incredible benefits of this ancient remedy.

By now, you've likely discovered how castor oil can reduce inflammation, boost wellness, and rejuvenate your skin—all using nature's wisdom instead of modern chemicals.

This book was written for people like you, who are searching for holistic, natural alternatives to chemical-laden solutions. I hope the practical tips and recipes have inspired you to take charge of your health and beauty in a more mindful way.

If you're finding value in this book, I would love to hear your thoughts. Reviews on Amazon make a huge difference in helping others discover this natural alternative.

Simply go to the book's page on Amazon, scroll down to the "Write a Customer Review" button, and share your experience.

Even a few sentences about what you've learned or found helpful would mean the world to me and to others searching for this knowledge.

Thank you for being part of this journey!

Barbara

Chapter 6
Holistic Health and Lifestyle Integration

Imagine a peaceful morning, the sun peeking through the curtains, casting a warm glow across your yoga mat. The air is filled with the subtle, comforting aroma of castor oil, creating a serene environment perfect for starting your day with intention. In the backdrop of modern life's hustle, incorporating castor oil into your yoga and meditation practices can transform your routine into a holistic experience. This chapter explores how castor oil can deepen your physical practice and enhance your mental clarity, creating a bridge between ancient wisdom and contemporary wellness.

6.1 Incorporating Castor Oil into Yoga and Meditation Practices

Yoga is a practice that unites the body and mind, promoting flexibility, strength, and inner peace. Integrating castor oil into your yoga routine can amplify these benefits by preparing your body for movement. Before you unroll your mat, consider using castor oil as a massage oil to warm your muscles. Its rich, viscous texture penetrates deeply, offering a soothing warmth that prepares your muscles for the asanas ahead. This pre-yoga massage not only prevents injuries but also enhances your flexibility, allowing for a deeper stretch and more fluid movement. Applying castor oil to your joints can further increase flexibility, reducing stiffness and easing tension. This simple addition to your routine can transform your practice, making each pose more comfortable and accessible.

Transitioning from physical movement to stillness, castor oil can also enrich your meditation practice. Its subtle, earthy aroma serves as a calming agent, helping to center your thoughts and deepen your focus. As you settle into meditation, the scent of castor oil envelops you, creating a tranquil atmosphere that encourages mindfulness. This aromatic presence acts as a gentle reminder to return to your breath whenever your mind begins to wander. Moreover, castor oil can play a role in grounding rituals, providing a tactile connection to the present moment. By anointing your hands with castor oil before meditation, you engage your senses, fostering a connection between mind and body that supports a more profound meditative state.

To fully integrate castor oil into your yoga and meditation practices, consider these practical steps.

- Start with a simple recipe for a yoga mat cleaning spray: Combine castor oil with water and a few drops of your favorite essential oil, such as lavender or eucalyptus. This natural spray not only cleanses your mat but also leaves behind a soothing scent, enhancing your practice from the ground up.

- For a pre-meditation hand ritual, warm a small amount of castor oil between your palms, then gently massage your hands, focusing on each finger and joint. This ritual not only prepares your body for stillness but also becomes a moment of self-care, grounding you in the present and readying you for meditation.

Yoga practitioners and meditation guides alike have shared their experiences with incorporating castor oil into their routines. One yoga instructor noted how using castor oil as a massage oil before class enhanced her students' flexibility, allowing them to achieve deeper poses with ease. Another meditation guide spoke of the transformative power of castor oil's scent, describing it as a gentle anchor that brings focus and clarity during meditation. These testimonials highlight the synergy between castor oil and mindfulness practices, underscoring its potential to elevate your routine.

Reflection Section: Personalizing Your Practice

Take a moment to reflect on your current yoga and meditation practices. How might incorporating castor oil enhance your experience? Consider setting an intention for your practice, whether it's to deepen your stretches, find greater focus, or simply enjoy a moment of self-care. Write down your thoughts and plan how you might introduce castor oil into your routine, personalizing its use to fit your unique needs.

6.2 Balancing Chakras: Energetic Uses of Castor Oil

Imagine the body as a complex network of energy centers, known as chakras. These centers, according to Eastern traditions, play a crucial role in maintaining physical and emotional health. Chakras, often visualized as spinning wheels of energy, interact with your body's vital functions and emotional states. Each of the seven primary chakras corresponds to specific physical, emotional, and spiritual aspects. When these chakras are balanced, energy flows freely, promoting overall well-being. However, blockages or imbalances can lead to a range of issues, from stress to physical ailments. Here, castor oil emerges as a gentle yet potent tool for energy healing, helping to restore harmony within this intricate system.

Applying castor oil in chakra work can facilitate a deeper connection to your energetic self. Start by using castor oil on the forehead, directly over the third eye chakra, also known as Ajna. This chakra is associated with intuition and perception, guiding your wisdom and insight. Massaging a small amount of castor oil here can aid in opening this energy center, enhancing your intuitive capabilities. The oil serves as a conduit, encouraging energy flow and helping to dissolve any blockages that may hinder your perception and clarity. Another application involves the heart chakra, or Anahata, which governs love and compassion. Combining castor oil with floral essential oils, such as rose or jasmine, can create an aromatic blend that opens this chakra, fostering a sense of emotional balance and empathy. This blend not only nurtures your emotional well-being but also invites a harmonious connection with others.

Balanced chakras can lead to significant improvements in your overall wellness. Emotionally, you may notice a newfound stability, where reactions become more measured and responses more thoughtful. Clarity of mind often accompanies this balance, allowing for better decision-making and a more profound understanding of your life's path. On a spiritual level, balanced chakras enhance awareness, fostering a deeper connection with the universe and a greater sense of purpose. This heightened spiritual awareness can bring about a peaceful state of being, where the noise of everyday life quiets and a calm, centered presence takes its place. The benefits of balanced chakras are holistic, positively affecting both your inner and outer worlds.

To support chakra alignment, consider establishing a ritual that incorporates castor oil.

- Begin with a chakra-balancing bath, designed to cleanse and energize your body.

- Add a few tablespoons of castor oil to a warm bath, along with Epsom salts and a handful of dried lavender.

- As you soak, visualize each chakra opening and spinning freely, releasing tension and inviting positivity. This ritual not only detoxifies your body but also invigorates your energy centers, leaving you refreshed and recharged.

- Complementing this bath, guided visualization exercises with castor oil can further deepen your practice.

- Sit comfortably and apply a small amount of castor oil to your palms.

- Close your eyes and imagine a vibrant energy flowing from your hands to each chakra, balancing and harmonizing them. As you move through each energy center, visualize its color and feel its unique vibration, reinforcing the connection between your physical and energetic bodies.

The practice of balancing chakras with castor oil is rooted in both ancient wisdom and modern understanding. It offers a tangible way to engage with your energetic health, transforming abstract concepts into meaningful rituals. As you explore these practices, you'll find that castor oil serves as a versatile ally, supporting your journey toward balance and harmony. Whether through targeted applications or immersive rituals, the potential for growth and healing is vast, limited only by your willingness to explore and embrace the energies within.

6.3 Castor Oil in Aromatherapy: Blends for Mindfulness

Imagine the gentle waft of soothing scents enveloping your senses, creating an oasis of calm in your daily life. Castor oil plays a unique role in aromatherapy, serving as a carrier oil that enhances the diffusion and longevity of essential oils. Its thick consistency allows for a slow, steady release of fragrance, ensuring that the calming or invigorating effects of your chosen oils linger longer. This compatibility with essential oils makes castor oil an ideal medium for creating personalized aromatherapy blends that cater to your specific needs.

One popular blend for mental clarity and relaxation combines lavender and chamomile. To create this calming blend, simply mix a tablespoon of castor oil with ten drops of lavender essential oil and five drops of chamomile essential oil. This concoction can be used in a diffuser, filling your space with a tranquil scent that promotes relaxation and eases stress. For a more invigorating experience, consider a citrus and mint mixture. Combine castor oil with five drops of grapefruit essential oil and five drops of peppermint essential oil. This blend not only refreshes the senses but also enhances focus, making it perfect for moments when you need a mental boost.

Aromatherapy has long been celebrated for its positive impact on mental well-being. The right blend of scents can significantly reduce stress and anxiety, turning ordinary moments into opportunities for mindfulness and reflection. As the soothing aromas of lavender and chamomile fill the air, stress seems to melt away, replaced by a sense of peace and calm. These scents have been shown to lower cortisol levels, the hormone associated with stress, allowing you to relax more deeply. On the other hand, the invigorating properties of citrus and mint can sharpen your focus and clarity, making it easier to concentrate on tasks and maintain a steady flow of productivity.

Creating a mindful environment with castor oil blends is a simple yet effective way to enhance your daily life. Diffusing these blends in your workspace can help maintain focus and alleviate stress during work or study sessions. The steady release of scent from castor oil ensures a consistent atmosphere, free from the need for constant replenishment. Scented sachets infused with your favorite blend can be placed in meditation spaces or under your pillow, subtly enhancing your environment with calming fragrances. This gentle aroma can be a constant companion in your pursuit of mindfulness, providing an anchor for your thoughts and a cue to return to the present moment.

To get the most out of your aromatherapy experience, consider these tips. First, select high-quality essential oils that align with your goals, whether relaxation, focus, or energy. Pair them with pure castor oil, ensuring the blend remains stable and effective. Experiment with different ratios to find the perfect balance for your needs. Remember to rotate scents periodically to avoid olfactory fatigue, which can diminish their impact over time. And finally, create a dedicated space for aromatherapy, a place where you can retreat, even for a few minutes, to center yourself amidst the demands of daily life. This intentional use of scent can transform ordinary moments into meaningful rituals, fostering a deeper connection to your environment and well-being.

6.4 Creating Daily Rituals: Mindful Living with Castor Oil

In our fast-paced lives, establishing daily rituals becomes a sanctuary for mental health. These rituals anchor us, creating moments of intentional living that cultivate awareness and promote consistency in our wellness routines. Incorporating castor oil into these daily practices can deepen your mindfulness, transforming simple actions into meaningful experiences. Imagine starting your day with a castor oil self-massage. This ritual not only awakens your senses but also encourages a deep connection with your body. As you gently massage the oil into your skin, notice its texture and warmth. This moment of focus allows you to center yourself before the day unfolds, setting a mindful tone that carries you through the hours ahead.

Evenings offer another opportunity to integrate castor oil into your routine. Consider a relaxing foot bath to unwind after a long day. Fill a basin with warm water and add a few drops of castor oil, along with your favorite calming essential oils like lavender or chamomile. As you soak your feet, let the stress of the day melt away. This simple act can transform your evening into a ritual of relaxation, promoting a restful night's sleep. The consistency of these practices reinforces positive habits, grounding you in self-care, and creating a sense of order amidst life's chaos.

Establishing structured rituals with castor oil can profoundly impact your well-being. These routines provide a framework that nurtures both mental and physical health, fostering a sense of calm and balance. By dedicating time each day to these mindful practices, you reinforce a commitment to yourself, prioritizing your health and happiness. Over time, these rituals become second nature, seamlessly integrating into your life and nurturing your well-being from the inside out.

Personal stories and cultural traditions provide rich examples of how castor oil has been woven into daily life around the world. In

India, for instance, castor oil has long been used in the ayurvedic practice of Abhyanga, a daily self-massage ritual that enhances circulation and promotes detoxification. This tradition emphasizes the importance of nurturing the body through regular touch, using the oil as a conduit for healing and balance. Similarly, in the Caribbean, castor oil is often incorporated into hair care routines, with mothers and grandmothers passing down the tradition of weekly oil treatments to maintain healthy, lustrous hair.

In my own experience, integrating castor oil into my daily rituals has been transformative. I remember a particularly stressful period in my life when I began a nightly foot bath routine with castor oil. This simple act of self-care became a cherished ritual, offering a moment of peace and reflection each evening. Over time, I noticed a profound shift in my mental state. The consistency of this practice provided a sense of stability and comfort, helping me navigate challenges with greater ease and resilience. These personal anecdotes and cultural practices highlight the universal appeal of castor oil as a tool for daily wellness, offering a timeless connection to self-care that transcends borders and generations.

As you explore the potential of castor oil in your own life, consider how these rituals might enhance your daily routine. Whether through a morning massage or an evening soak, these practices offer a chance to reconnect with yourself, fostering mindfulness and promoting well-being. By embracing these rituals, you invite a sense of intentionality and calm into your life, nurturing your mind and body in harmony with nature's wisdom.

Incorporating these rituals not only nurtures the body but also enriches the soul. As we move forward, exploring further how castor oil can be part of a sustainable lifestyle, you'll discover even more ways this humble oil can transform daily living. From personal care to environmental consciousness, castor oil continues to reveal its versatile benefits, inviting you to deepen your connection with yourself and the world around you.

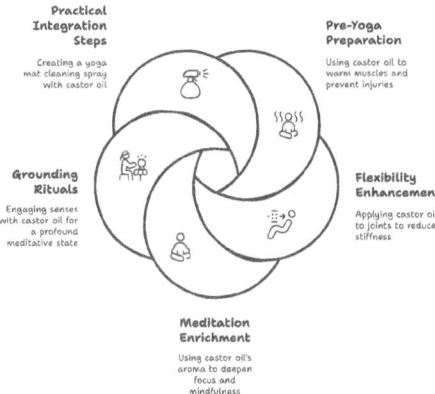

Chapter 7
Addressing Common Concerns and Missteps

When you first pick up a bottle of castor oil, you might see it as a simple remedy with a long history. Yet, like any powerful tool, it requires respect and understanding to use effectively. Imagine a world where every drop of this golden elixir enhances your life without a single misstep. To achieve this, it's essential to address common concerns and avoid potential pitfalls that can turn your castor oil experience from beneficial to bothersome. This chapter will guide you through essential safety measures, ensuring that your journey with castor oil is as smooth and rewarding as possible.

7.1 Safe Use Guidelines: Avoiding Common Pitfalls

Navigating the safe use of castor oil begins with understanding its potent nature. While it offers numerous benefits, ingesting large quantities can lead to unpleasant side effects like digestive distress or dehydration. The main component, ricinoleic acid, is powerful in small doses (SOURCE 1). However, when consumed excessively, it can upset the body's delicate balance, leading to electrolyte disturbances. To prevent this, always adhere to recommended dosages and consider professional guidance, especially if you're new to using castor oil internally.

Handling and storing castor oil safely is just as crucial. Store it in a cool, dark place, away from direct sunlight and heat sources. This not only preserves its quality but also prevents any potential degradation that could reduce its effectiveness. If you're transferring the oil to a different container, ensure it's clean and preferably made of glass, as plastic can leach chemicals into the oil. Handling the oil with clean hands or tools also minimizes the risk of contamination, keeping your castor oil pure and safe to use.

Before applying castor oil extensively to your skin, it's wise to perform a patch test. This simple step can help you avoid allergic reactions, which can include symptoms like redness, itching, or swelling (SOURCE 2). To conduct a patch test, apply a small amount of castor oil to a discreet area of your skin, such as the inside of your elbow. Leave it for 24 hours and monitor for any adverse reactions. If you notice any irritation, it might be best to avoid using the oil or consult a healthcare professional for advice. This precaution is particularly important for those with sensitive skin or a history of allergies.

The quality of your castor oil plays a pivotal role in its safety and effectiveness. Using low-quality or adulterated oils can introduce contaminants that compromise the oil's benefits and potentially harm your skin. Always choose reputable brands known for their commitment to purity and quality. Look for certifications, such as USDA Organic, which assure you of the oil's authenticity and safety. Reputable brands often provide transparency about their sourcing and production processes, giving you confidence in your choice.

When applying castor oil topically, exercise caution to ensure safe use. Avoid applying it near your eyes, as its thick consistency can cause irritation. If you do get some in your eyes, rinse immediately with plenty of water. For optimal benefits, cleanse the area thoroughly before and after application. This not only enhances the oil's absorption but also prevents any buildup that could clog pores or irritate the skin. By maintaining these practices, you ensure that your use of castor oil remains beneficial and trouble-free.

Reflection Section: Your Castor Oil Safety Checklist

- **Ingestion Precautions:**

Confirm you've reviewed recommended dosages and consulted with a healthcare provider if needed.

- **Storage Best Practices:**

Ensure your castor oil is stored in a cool, dark place, in a clean glass container.

- **Patch Testing:**

Perform a patch test and monitor for any reactions before extensive use.

- **Quality Assurance:**

Verify the oil's brand reputation and look for quality certifications.

- **Topical Application Care:**

Avoid eye contact and cleanse the skin thoroughly post-application.

By following these safety guidelines, you create a solid foundation for incorporating castor oil into your life, maximizing its benefits while minimizing potential risks. As you continue exploring the myriad uses of castor oil, keep these practices in mind, ensuring each application is as safe and effective as possible.

7.2 Dosage and Application: Getting It Right Every Time

Understanding the correct dosage of castor oil is vital to tapping into its benefits without encountering any pitfalls. Whether you're using it for its internal or external advantages, getting the dosage right can make all the difference. For internal use, the recommended dosage for adults ranges from 15 to 60 milliliters per day, depending on the desired effect and individual tolerance. For children, the dosage should be significantly reduced; a safe starting point is usually between 5 to 15 milliliters, tailored to their age and specific needs. It's crucial to remember that these are general guidelines, and consulting with a healthcare professional can provide personalized advice that considers individual health conditions and other medications.

When it comes to external application, using the right amount of castor oil can optimize its effectiveness while minimizing waste. For hair treatments, a small amount, typically around a teaspoon, is sufficient to cover medium-length hair. Starting at the scalp, gently massage the oil in circular motions to stimulate blood flow and enhance absorption. This technique not only promotes hair growth but also ensures the oil penetrates deeply, nourishing the hair from root to tip. For skin treatments, a few drops are usually enough to cover a specific area. Use gentle, upward strokes to apply the oil, which helps lift and firm the skin. This method allows the oil to absorb slowly, delivering its moisturizing properties without leaving a greasy residue.

Timing and frequency play a crucial role in maximizing the benefits of castor oil. Applying it at night can yield the best results as the body enters a rest and repair mode during sleep. This timing allows the oil to work in harmony with your body's natural processes, enhancing its effects on both skin and hair. For those with dry skin, daily application may be beneficial, providing continuous hydration and protection. Conversely, individuals with oily skin might find a weekly application sufficient to maintain balance without overloading the skin with extra moisture. Adjusting the frequency based on your skin type ensures you reap the benefits without causing any imbalance.

Visual aids can significantly enhance the understanding of correct application techniques. Imagine a diagram showing the precise areas for optimal application, such as the scalp for hair growth or the under-eye area for reducing puffiness. Step-by-step illustrations can guide you through the process, from warming the oil in your hands to using the right massaging motions. These visuals not only clarify the technique but also serve as a handy reference, ensuring you can apply castor oil with confidence and precision. While this book format doesn't allow for actual illustrations, consider seeking out resources or tutorials that provide these visual guides to supplement your understanding.

With these detailed insights into dosage and application, you can better integrate castor oil into your routine, maximizing its benefits while avoiding common missteps. Whether you're using it for internal or external purposes, the key lies in understanding your body's unique needs and adjusting accordingly. It's about finding the balance that works for you, allowing castor oil to enhance your health and beauty naturally.

7.3 Combining Castor Oil with Other Natural Remedies

When exploring natural remedies, combining castor oil with other products can amplify its benefits, creating powerful synergies that enhance overall well-being. To ensure compatibility and avoid unwanted interactions, it's important to check ingredient labels and understand how different substances react with each other. Some ingredients may not work well together, causing irritation or diminishing each other's effects. It's a bit like cooking; some flavors blend beautifully, while others clash. Keeping an eye out for known allergens or irritants in other products is a good start. For tailored advice, consulting with a healthcare provider can be invaluable, especially if you have sensitive skin or specific health concerns.

Consider the soothing power of combining castor oil with aloe vera for skin treatments. Aloe vera is renowned for its cooling and anti-inflammatory properties, which complement the moisturizing and healing capabilities of castor oil. When mixed, these two create a potent balm that can soothe sunburns, calm irritated skin, and even help with minor cuts and abrasions. Mixing them is simple: blend equal parts of castor oil and aloe vera gel until you achieve a smooth consistency. This mixture offers a gentle, natural remedy that cools and hydrates, leaving your skin feeling refreshed and rejuvenated.

For hair care, castor oil pairs beautifully with coconut oil, a duo that hydrates and strengthens hair. Coconut oil penetrates the hair shaft, providing deep conditioning, while castor oil forms a protective layer on the hair surface, locking in moisture. This combination can help reduce breakage, add shine, and encourage healthy hair growth. To create a hair mask, mix one part castor oil with two parts coconut oil, warm it slightly to enhance absorption, and apply generously from roots to tips. Leave it in for at least an hour, or overnight for a more intensive treatment, before washing it out thoroughly.

Understanding individual responses is crucial when using natural remedies. Skin sensitivity varies greatly from person to person, so what works for one individual may not be suitable for another. Pay attention to how your skin reacts to new combinations and adjust the ratios or try different pairings if needed. For instance, if you find the mix of castor oil and coconut oil too heavy for your hair, consider reducing the amount of castor oil or adding a lighter oil, like jojoba, to balance the blend. Personal experience and experimentation are key to finding what works best for your unique needs.

Integrating castor oil with other natural remedies can support overall wellness by creating comprehensive routines that address multiple aspects of health. By thoughtfully combining these natural ingredients, you can design personalized wellness regimens that cater to your specific goals, whether it's achieving clear skin, strong hair, or improved relaxation. The synergistic effects of these combinations can enhance your body's natural healing processes, offering a holistic approach to health that is both effective and nurturing. This method of blending remedies encourages a balanced lifestyle, where natural products work together to support your well-being, just as different elements of nature coexist harmoniously.

Creating a routine that incorporates various natural remedies allows you to address multiple health goals simultaneously. For instance, you might start your day with a soothing castor oil and aloe vera face mask, then apply a coconut oil and castor oil hair treatment before bed. Over time, these practices can become a comforting ritual that not only enhances your physical health but also provides a moment of peace and self-care in your daily life. This holistic approach to wellness emphasizes the interconnectedness of mind and body, promoting a sense of balance and harmony that extends beyond the physical benefits of the remedies themselves.

Interactive Element: Personalized Remedy Journal

Keeping a journal can help you track your experiences with different combinations of castor oil and other natural remedies. Note

THE HIDDEN POWER OF CASTOR OIL: NATURE'S...   75

the ingredients used, the ratios, the method of application, and, most importantly, how your skin or hair responds. Over time, this journal will become a valuable resource, guiding you in refining your personal wellness routine. It encourages mindfulness and reflection, allowing you to make informed adjustments based on your observations. Recording your journey with natural remedies can also highlight the progress you make, reinforcing the positive impact these practices have on your life.

7.4 Recognizing and Managing Adverse Reactions

As you embrace the many benefits of castor oil, it's important to remain vigilant for any adverse reactions your body might have. Recognizing these reactions early can prevent minor issues from becoming more serious. One of the most common signs is skin irritation, which can manifest as redness, itching, or a rash. This may occur if your skin is sensitive or if the oil is applied too liberally. Digestive discomfort is another potential reaction, especially if castor oil is ingested in larger amounts than recommended. Symptoms can include stomach cramps, nausea, or diarrhea, which reflect the body's response to the oil's potent laxative effects (SOURCE 1). Understanding these signs allows you to act quickly, ensuring that your experience with castor oil remains positive.

If you notice any mild reactions, taking immediate steps can mitigate discomfort. The first and most crucial action is to discontinue use. Give your body a chance to recuperate without further exposure to the irritant. If skin irritation occurs, applying a soothing agent like aloe vera can help calm the affected area. Aloe vera is renowned for its anti-inflammatory properties, which can reduce redness and provide relief from itching (SOURCE 3). Gently apply a small amount to the irritated skin, and let it absorb naturally. For digestive discomfort, hydrating with plenty of water helps flush out the system, aiding recovery. If symptoms persist, consider seeking medical advice to rule out any underlying issues.

Knowing when to consult a healthcare provider is key to managing more severe reactions. Persistent or severe symptoms, such as continuous skin irritation that doesn't improve with home remedies, warrant professional attention. Similarly, if you experience significant allergic responses like swelling, hives, or difficulty breathing, seek medical assistance immediately. These could indicate a more serious allergy that requires intervention (SOURCE 2). Consulting a healthcare provider ensures that you receive appropriate treatment and guidance tailored to your specific needs. They can also help determine whether castor oil is suitable for your skin type or if alternative remedies might be better suited.

Preventing future adverse reactions involves a thoughtful approach to reintroducing castor oil into your routine. Start by using it sparingly, applying a small amount to a less sensitive area, and carefully monitoring your body's response. Gradual reintroduction allows you to gauge tolerance and adjust usage accordingly. If previous reactions were severe, consider trying alternative forms or products. For instance, choosing a version of castor oil that is specifically formulated for sensitive skin might reduce the risk of irritation. Alternatively, you might explore products that combine castor oil with other soothing ingredients, providing a gentler application.

Reintroducing castor oil after an adverse event requires patience and mindfulness. Keep a journal to track any reactions, noting what works and what doesn't. This practice not only helps refine your approach but also empowers you to make informed decisions about your health and wellness. By understanding your body's unique needs, you can tailor your use of castor oil to maximize benefits while minimizing risks. This balanced approach ensures that you continue to enjoy the myriad advantages castor oil offers, without compromising your comfort or peace of mind.

In navigating the world of natural remedies, awareness and education are your allies. Recognizing potential reactions and taking proactive steps to manage them ensures that your journey with castor oil is both safe and rewarding. With careful attention and thoughtful practice, you can harness the full potential of this versatile oil, enhancing your health and well-being in harmony with nature's gifts. As you continue to explore the possibilities of castor oil, remember that knowledge and consideration are your best tools for success.

Safe and Effective Use of Castor Oil

- Ingestion Precautions
  - Recommended Dosages
  - Professional Guidance
- Handling and Storage
  - Cool, Dark Place
  - Clean Containers
- Quality Assurance
  - Reputable Brands
  - Certifications
- Patch Testing
  - Allergy Symptoms
  - Testing Procedure
- Topical Application
  - Avoid Eye Contact
  - Cleanse Before/After

(Castor Oil Safety)

Chapter 8
Sustainability and Environmental Impact

Picture a world where every product we use contributes to the health of our planet. It may seem like a distant dream, but with industries like castor oil leading the charge, it's closer than you think. Castor oil, a humble yet powerful natural resource, is at the forefront of a shift toward sustainable practices. This shift isn't just a trend; it's a necessary evolution. As consumers, our choices can either support this movement or hinder it. Understanding the impact of sustainable sourcing in the castor oil industry is crucial for making informed decisions that align with environmental goals.

Sustainable sourcing practices are pivotal in the castor oil industry, contributing significantly to environmental health. These practices aim to minimize the carbon footprint by prioritizing local sourcing. When oil is produced and consumed locally, it reduces the need for extensive transportation, which in turn cuts down on carbon emissions. This not only benefits the environment but also supports local economies by keeping profits within the community. Additionally, sustainable sourcing encourages biodiversity in farming regions. Castor plants, when cultivated responsibly, can coexist with other crops, fostering a biodiverse ecosystem that supports various forms of life. This biodiversity is essential for maintaining ecological balance and ensuring the resilience of agricultural systems against pests and diseases.

Transparency and traceability are key elements in ethical sourcing. They provide consumers with the information needed to make responsible choices. Certification labels such as Fair Trade and Organic are more than just stamps of approval; they are assurances of quality and ethics. These labels indicate that the product meets strict environmental and social standards. Fair Trade, for instance, ensures that farmers receive fair wages and work under safe conditions, while Organic certification confirms that the product is free from harmful chemicals. Brand transparency regarding sourcing locations further builds trust. When companies openly share where and how their castor oil is sourced, they demonstrate a commitment to ethical practices and allow consumers to verify the product's authenticity.

Identifying eco-friendly brands requires a discerning eye and a commitment to sustainability. Consumers can evaluate brands by examining their commitment to sustainable agriculture practices. This includes using organic farming methods that prioritize soil health and reduce chemical inputs. Brands should also engage in fair labor practices, ensuring that workers are treated with dignity and respect. These practices not only improve the quality of the product but also contribute to social equity. By choosing brands that prioritize sustainability and fair labor, consumers support a more just and environmentally friendly industry.

Case studies of exemplary sustainable brands provide real-world examples of success in the industry. For instance, the Castor Model Farm Project in India is a beacon of innovation and sustainability (SOURCE 2). This project works to improve the profitability and sustainability of castor farming by enhancing yield and reducing input costs. It serves as a model for other regions, demonstrating the potential for sustainable practices to transform the industry. Another example is Acme-Hardesty, a major distributor of castor oil that partners with sustainability initiatives to promote environmentally friendly practices (SOURCE 2). These companies are not only leading in sustainability but also creating positive community impacts through various projects. They show that it is possible to balance profitability with environmental responsibility.

Checklist for Choosing Eco-Friendly Brands

- **Local Sourcing**:

Does the brand prioritize local production to reduce carbon emissions?

- **Biodiversity Support**:

Are farming practices promoting a biodiverse ecosystem?

- **Certification Labels**:

Look for Fair Trade and Organic certifications for assurance of ethical practices.

- **Transparency**:

Does the brand provide detailed information about sourcing locations?

- **Sustainable Agriculture**:

Check for organic farming methods and reduced chemical use.

- **Fair Labor Practices**:

Ensure the brand engages in practices that respect and support workers.

By integrating these criteria into your purchasing decisions, you can support brands that are making a positive impact on the planet. This not only enhances your personal well-being but also contributes to a more sustainable future for everyone. Choosing eco-friendly brands is a powerful way to align your values with your consumption habits, paving the way for a healthier world.

8.1 Castor Oil and Environmental Stewardship

Environmental stewardship is about taking responsibility for our planet and nurturing its resources for future generations. It's a philosophy that aligns perfectly with the production and use of castor oil. By reducing chemical inputs through organic farming, the castor oil industry sets a benchmark for ecological balance. Traditional farming often relies heavily on synthetic fertilizers and pesticides, which can harm soil health and biodiversity. However, organic farming methods used in castor oil production avoid these chemicals, instead focusing on natural alternatives that nourish the soil. This approach not only maintains the integrity of the soil but actively encourages its regeneration. Healthy soil is the foundation of a vibrant ecosystem, supporting plant growth and the myriad organisms that call the soil home.

The ecological benefits of castor oil plants extend far beyond the farm. These plants are naturally drought-resistant, making them ideal for areas with limited water resources. Their ability to thrive with minimal water reduces the strain on local water supplies, conserving this precious resource for other uses. Additionally, the deep root systems of castor oil plants contribute to soil stabilization and erosion control. In areas prone to erosion, these roots anchor the soil, preventing it from being washed away by rain or wind. This not only preserves the land but also protects waterways from sediment pollution. The presence of castor oil plants in agricultural landscapes can thus play a vital role in maintaining ecological balance and enhancing the resilience of ecosystems.

In sustainable agriculture, castor oil holds a unique position as both a crop and a tool. Its use as a natural pest deterrent is particularly noteworthy. The ricin present in castor oil seeds deters a wide range of pests, reducing the need for synthetic pesticides. Farmers can plant castor oil alongside other crops, using it as a natural barrier against insects. This integration into crop rotation and polyculture systems enhances biodiversity and soil health. Polyculture, the practice of growing multiple crops together, mimics natural ecosystems and can lead to improved yields and pest resistance. Castor oil's role in these systems highlights its versatility and value in promoting sustainable farming practices.

Initiatives that promote environmental stewardship in the castor oil industry are gaining momentum. Partnerships between NGOs and castor oil producers are driving change by supporting sustainable practices and improving the livelihoods of farmers. These collaborations often focus on education, providing farmers with the knowledge they need to implement environmentally friendly techniques. Educational programs are vital in this regard, offering training on sustainable farming methods and resource management. By empowering farmers with the skills to cultivate castor oil sustainably, these programs ensure that the benefits extend beyond environmental health to social and economic well-being.

Such efforts demonstrate that sustainability is not just an environmental issue but a holistic one, encompassing economic viability and social equity. As more stakeholders recognize the potential of castor oil to support ecological balance, the industry is poised to become a model of environmental stewardship. The continued success of these initiatives depends on the collective action of producers, consumers, and policymakers, each playing a crucial role in shaping a sustainable future.

8.2 The Role of Castor Oil in Zero Waste Living

Imagine a lifestyle where waste is a thing of the past. This is the vision behind the zero waste philosophy. At its core, zero waste living is about minimizing what we discard and maximizing what we reuse. It's a commitment to living in a way that reduces our environmental footprint. Castor oil plays a surprisingly pivotal role in this lifestyle. Its versatility means it can replace many single-use products, reducing the need for plastic packaging and promoting sustainability. By using castor oil, you can cut down on wasteful habits, one product at a time.

When you choose products with minimal packaging, you actively support the zero waste movement. Castor oil is often packaged in recyclable or reusable containers, which aligns perfectly with zero waste principles. By selecting products in glass bottles or refillable options, you eliminate the need for constant repurchasing of plastic bottles. This simple choice has a ripple effect, reducing the amount of waste that ends up in landfills. Consider the impact of replacing a single-use plastic cleaner with a DIY solution made from castor oil. Not only do you save money, but you also reduce your household's plastic waste, contributing positively to the environment.

Castor oil's role in zero waste living extends beyond its packaging. Its multifunctional nature allows it to replace multiple products in your home. For instance, you can create a range of DIY household cleaners using castor oil as a base. These cleaners effectively replace single-use chemical products that often come in non-recyclable packaging. By mixing castor oil with other natural ingredients like vinegar and baking soda, you can make powerful yet eco-friendly cleaning solutions. These DIY cleaners work wonders on everything from kitchen counters to bathroom tiles, proving that a single bottle of castor oil can serve countless purposes.

The impact of castor oil-based products on waste reduction is significant. Many beauty and personal care items made with castor oil come in biodegradable formulations. These products not only nourish your skin and hair but also break down naturally, leaving no trace behind. By switching to castor oil-based beauty products, you reduce the need for multiple items, each with its own packaging. This simplification of your routine aligns with zero waste goals, as it encourages the use of fewer, more sustainable products. Moreover, the natural properties of castor oil mean that these products are kind to your skin and the planet.

To incorporate castor oil into your zero waste routine, start by making bulk purchases. Buying in larger quantities reduces packaging waste and often results in cost savings. Store your castor oil in a cool, dark place to maintain its quality over time. You can also participate in local zero waste communities to exchange tips and resources. These communities often host events where members share bulk purchases or swap reusable containers. By getting involved, you can learn more about sustainable living and connect with others who share your commitment to reducing waste.

Interactive Element: DIY Cleaner Recipe

Try making your own all-purpose cleaner using castor oil. You will need:

- 1 cup water

- 1 cup white vinegar

- 1 tablespoon castor oil

- 10 drops of lemon essential oil (optional)

Mix all ingredients in a spray bottle and shake well. Use this cleaner on countertops, sinks, and other surfaces. By using this DIY cleaner, you reduce reliance on chemical products and contribute to a zero waste lifestyle.

Incorporating castor oil into your zero waste living not only benefits the environment but also simplifies your life. By focusing on products that are multifunctional and sustainably packaged, you create a home that reflects your values. Each small change you make has the potential to inspire others, fostering a community of individuals committed to a waste-free future. Embracing zero waste principles with castor oil is a step toward a cleaner, healthier planet.

8.3 Green Beauty: Eco-Conscious Personal Care Choices

Imagine standing in front of a shelf filled with beauty products, each claiming to enhance your skin or hair in miraculous ways. But in the world of green beauty, the focus shifts from mere aesthetics to a more profound commitment to health and sustainability. Green beauty embodies an approach where products are crafted without harmful chemicals and synthetic ingredients. Instead, they embrace the power of nature, utilizing renewable and biodegradable components that nourish both you and the environment. In this way, green beauty aligns with the ideals of eco-conscious living, offering solutions that care for the planet as much as they care for you.

Castor oil shines brightly in the realm of green beauty, offering a natural alternative to synthetic emollients. Its rich, moisturizing properties make it an excellent base for a variety of personal care products. Whether used in lotions, creams, or balms, castor oil provides deep hydration, leaving skin soft and supple without the need for artificial additives. Its versatility extends beyond skincare, finding a place in haircare formulations as well. Castor oil's thick consistency and nourishing qualities make it perfect for conditioning treatments, serums, and even shampoos. It helps tame frizz, promote shine, and support healthy hair growth, all while maintaining a commitment to natural ingredients.

When selecting eco-friendly personal care products, it's important to become an informed consumer. Start by reading labels carefully for eco-certifications and natural ingredients. Look for products that bear certifications like USDA Organic or Ecocert, which ensure that the ingredients meet stringent environmental and health standards. These labels are not just marketing tools; they are guarantees of quality and safety. Additionally, consider the packaging. Brands that prioritize sustainable packaging initiatives demonstrate their dedication to reducing waste. Glass bottles, recycled materials, and minimal packaging are all indicators that a brand is committed to sustainability.

Several innovative brands are leading the charge in the world of green beauty, setting new standards for sustainability and effectiveness. For instance, EriCare, a leading brand in India, is known for its castor oil products that enhance hair, skin, and eyelashes naturally (SOURCE 4). Their commitment to clean beauty is evident in their product formulations, which avoid harmful chemicals and instead leverage the natural benefits of castor oil. Interviews with founders of such brands often reveal a deep passion for environmental impact and a desire to create products that are as kind to the earth as they are to the consumer. These pioneering companies are not just producing beauty items; they are crafting a movement that prioritizes the well-being of the planet.

In the pursuit of green beauty, it's crucial to support companies that align with these values. By choosing products from brands that focus on sustainability, you contribute to a larger effort to reduce environmental impact. This choice goes beyond individual benefit; it supports a collective move towards a more sustainable future. The beauty industry, long criticized for its environmental footprint, is undergoing a transformation, and castor oil is at the heart of this change. Its natural properties, combined with thoughtful, eco-friendly practices, make it a cornerstone of a beauty regimen that respects both the user and the planet.

As we explore the impact of castor oil in the context of green beauty, it's clear that every choice we make can contribute to a healthier, more sustainable world. The products we use daily are not just about personal care; they are about caring for the environment we inhabit. Embracing green beauty means embracing a lifestyle that values sustainability, health, and the intricate balance of our ecosystem. By integrating castor oil into your routine, you join a community of individuals committed to making a positive impact through conscious choices. This approach not only benefits your health but also sends a powerful message about the kind of future we want to build.

In the next chapter, we will delve into practical applications and recipes, showing how castor oil can be seamlessly integrated into everyday life. From beauty treatments to household solutions, the versatility of castor oil offers endless possibilities for enhancing both your well-being and your commitment to sustainability.

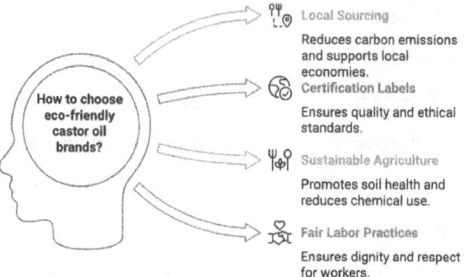

Chapter 9
Exploring Unique and Niche Uses

Imagine a sunny afternoon in your backyard, where your loyal companion frolics happily, free from the pesky fleas and ticks that often accompany warm weather. You've discovered a natural solution that not only keeps your furry friend comfortable but also supports their overall well-being. Castor oil, long esteemed for its health benefits in humans, holds a similar promise for our pets. This versatile oil, derived from the seeds of the Ricinus communis plant, offers a gentle yet effective approach to improving pet health and hygiene. Its applications in pet care extend beyond the ordinary, providing a holistic method for addressing common issues that our beloved animals face.

9.1 Castor Oil in Pet Care: Benefits and Precautions

In the realm of pet care, castor oil emerges as a valuable ally against fleas and ticks, those relentless critters that can turn a pleasant day into an itchy ordeal. When used as a natural repellent, castor oil creates an inhospitable environment for these pests without resorting to harsh chemicals. Its thick consistency allows it to adhere well to a pet's coat, forming a barrier that fleas and ticks find difficult to penetrate. This natural approach not only safeguards your pet but also offers peace of mind, knowing that you're using a safe, non-toxic solution to protect them.

The benefits of castor oil extend to soothing skin irritations and hot spots, common concerns for many pet owners. Hot spots, or acute moist dermatitis, are inflamed areas of skin that cause discomfort and persistent licking. Castor oil's anti-inflammatory properties help reduce redness and swelling while providing a protective layer that supports healing. When applied to the affected area, it calms irritation and promotes regeneration, offering relief to your pet and reducing the risk of further injury through scratching. Its moisturizing effect also helps prevent the skin from becoming dry and flaky, ensuring a healthier coat overall.

Dry, itchy skin is another prevalent issue among pets, leading to incessant scratching and discomfort. Castor oil's rich, emollient nature makes it an excellent moisturizer for easing this condition. By applying a diluted mixture of castor oil to your pet's skin, you can alleviate dryness and restore much-needed hydration. This not only soothes itching but also helps promote a shiny, healthy coat that reflects your pet's vitality. Regular application can transform your pet's coat, turning it from dull and lifeless to vibrant and glossy. The oil's natural nutrients support fur growth and improve texture, offering a holistic approach to maintaining your pet's external health.

When using castor oil on pets, safety is paramount. It's essential to dilute the oil with water or another carrier oil, such as coconut or olive oil, to ensure it's gentle enough for sensitive skin. A typical dilution ratio might be one part castor oil to four parts carrier oil, struck with the balance of effectiveness and safety. Apply this mixture sparingly, focusing on areas that require attention, such as spots with dry or irritated skin. Frequency depends on the condition being treated, but starting with one application per week allows you to monitor your pet's response and adjust as needed.

Despite its benefits, castor oil should be used with caution. Pets, curious by nature, may attempt to lick or ingest anything applied to their skin. As castor oil can act as a laxative if consumed in large amounts, it's crucial to prevent ingestion by your pet. Ensure that areas treated with castor oil are covered or inaccessible until the oil has absorbed. Additionally, monitor your pet for any signs of skin sensitivity or allergic reactions, such as redness or swelling, and consult a veterinarian if any adverse effects occur. While castor oil is generally safe, every pet is unique, and individual reactions can vary.

Incorporating castor oil into your pet care routine can be a rewarding experience, offering a natural, effective means of addressing common health concerns. By understanding the benefits and precautions associated with its use, you can ensure that your pet enjoys the best of what this remarkable oil has to offer. Whether soothing irritated skin or warding off unwanted pests, castor oil provides a gentle, holistic approach to enhancing your pet's quality of life. As you explore these applications, you'll find that castor oil is not just a remedy but a testament to the power of nature in caring for those we cherish.

9.2 Industrial Insights: Non-Toxic Household Solutions

Imagine walking into your home and breathing in air that feels clean and free of harsh chemical residues. This is the promise of non-toxic cleaning, and castor oil plays a significant role in achieving this healthy environment. Known for its moisturizing properties and gentle nature, castor oil offers a safe alternative to conventional chemical cleaners that often contain ingredients harmful to both health and the environment. Its versatility makes it an excellent choice for creating multi-purpose cleaning solutions that can tackle various surfaces throughout your home. Whether you're dealing with countertops, wooden furniture, or tile floors, castor oil can be combined with other natural ingredients to create effective cleaners that leave your space sparkling and fresh.

In the kitchen and bathroom, where grease and grime often accumulate, castor oil's natural degreasing properties come into play. Its thick consistency and ability to break down oils make it an ideal ingredient in cleaning solutions designed to cut through stubborn residues on stovetops, sinks, and tiles. Unlike harsh chemical degreasers that emit strong fumes and can irritate the skin and respiratory system, castor oil-based solutions offer a gentle yet powerful alternative. They lift away grease and dirt without leaving behind any toxic traces, contributing to a healthier indoor environment for you and your family.

For those interested in crafting their own eco-friendly cleaning products, a simple recipe for an all-purpose castor oil cleaner involves mixing equal parts of castor oil and white vinegar with a few drops of your favorite essential oil for fragrance. This mixture can be stored in a spray bottle and used on a variety of surfaces, from kitchen counters to bathroom fixtures. For glass and mirrors, a castor oil and vinegar glass cleaner can be made by combining one part castor oil with three parts vinegar and a splash of water. This formulation leaves glass surfaces streak-free and shiny, without the need for ammonia or other harsh chemicals typically found in commercial glass cleaners. These DIY solutions not only ensure a clean home but also align with sustainable living practices by reducing reliance on store-bought products and their associated packaging waste.

The environmental benefits of using non-toxic cleaning solutions like those made with castor oil are significant. Traditional cleaning products often contain chemicals that not only linger in the air but also contribute to indoor air pollution, affecting air quality and potentially impacting health over time. By opting for natural alternatives, you reduce the presence of these chemical residues in your home, creating a cleaner, more breathable environment. Furthermore, the runoff from cleaning products can enter waterways, causing harm to aquatic ecosystems. Non-toxic solutions mitigate this impact, as they break down more readily in the environment and pose less risk to wildlife and water quality.

To integrate castor oil into your sustainable home practices, consider using reusable cleaning cloths and tools. Microfiber cloths or reusable cotton pads work well with castor oil-based cleaners, reducing the need for disposable wipes and paper towels. This not only cuts down on waste but also enhances the cleaning process as these materials are designed to trap dust and dirt effectively. Adding essential oils to your cleaning solutions not only provides a pleasant aroma but also boosts the efficacy of the cleaners. Oils like lavender, tea tree, or lemon not only smell wonderful but also possess their own antibacterial and antifungal properties, complementing the cleaning power of castor oil.

Creating a non-toxic living environment with castor oil is more than just a cleaning choice; it represents a commitment to health, sustainability, and mindfulness in everyday practices. By embracing these natural solutions, you contribute to a healthier home and a cleaner planet. As you explore the potential of castor oil in household cleaning, you'll find that its benefits extend beyond hygiene, offering a path to a more eco-conscious lifestyle that respects both personal well-being and environmental health. This approach aligns with a growing awareness of the need to protect our planet and the desire to live in harmony with nature's offerings, using resources wisely and responsibly.

9.3 Artistic Applications: Using Castor Oil in Creative Projects

In the bustling studios of artists around the world, castor oil finds its place not just in health and beauty but as a subtle yet powerful medium in the realm of art. This versatile oil, known for its rich texture and gentle properties, has been embraced by creatives seeking to infuse their work with both innovation and sustainability. In oil painting, castor oil serves as an effective solvent, offering artists a non-toxic alternative to traditional turpentine or mineral spirits. Its unique consistency allows for the thinning of paints and adjusting viscosity, providing artists with greater control over texture and flow. This flexibility is particularly valuable when working on large canvases or intricate details, where the ability to manipulate the medium can transform a piece from ordinary to extraordinary.

Beyond its role as a solvent, castor oil acts as a base for homemade art supplies, expanding the possibilities for creativity. Artists can create their own paints, combining castor oil with natural pigments to develop custom hues and finishes. This not only fosters a deeper connection with the materials but also ensures that the resulting art is free from synthetic additives that can impact both the environment and the artist's health. Additionally, castor oil's natural properties make it an ideal component in the creation of natural dyes and inks. By blending it with plant-based pigments, artists can achieve vibrant, lasting colors that maintain their integrity over time. These natural inks offer a sustainable alternative to commercial products, reducing reliance on chemical-based dyes that often carry a significant environmental footprint.

In the hands of an artist, castor oil can also enhance the texture and gloss of a painting. When mixed with oil paints, it imparts a subtle sheen that brings depth and luminosity to the artwork. This gloss effect catches the light, adding a dynamic quality to the surface that can change with the viewer's perspective. It also allows for the creation of layered textures, where the oil's thickness can be manipulated to build up areas of interest and contrast. This versatility in application encourages experimentation, inviting artists to explore new techniques and push the boundaries of their creative expression. Whether used to achieve a smooth, polished finish or to accentuate the ruggedness of a landscape, castor oil fosters artistic exploration in ways that traditional materials may not.

Artists who have integrated castor oil into their work often speak of its impact not only on their art but also on their approach to sustainability. Many eco-conscious artists value castor oil for its non-toxic nature, which aligns with their commitment to reducing environmental harm. In interviews, these artists express appreciation for a medium that allows them to work without the health risks associated with conventional solvents. The ability to create in a safe, clean environment supports both their well-being and their artistic practice, allowing for longer, more productive work sessions without the concern of inhaling harmful fumes. Moreover, the use of castor oil supports a broader movement within the art community toward sustainable materials, reflecting a growing awareness of the need to balance creativity with environmental responsibility.

Case studies of innovative projects highlight the diverse applications of castor oil in art. One artist, inspired by the fluidity castor oil offers, developed a series of abstract works using a blend of castor oil and natural pigments. These pieces, characterized by their vibrant colors and flowing forms, evoke the organic movement of nature, marrying the artist's vision with the medium's inherent qualities. Another project focused on creating eco-friendly art installations, where castor oil was used to seal and protect large outdoor sculptures. Its weather-resistant properties ensured the longevity of the pieces, demonstrating castor oil's practical benefits in preserving art exposed to the elements. These projects not only showcase the artistic potential of castor oil but also underscore its role in fostering sustainable practices within the creative arts.

Incorporating castor oil into artistic endeavors offers a refreshing perspective on how traditional materials can be reimagined for modern use. Its adaptability and gentle impact make it an appealing choice for artists committed to innovation and sustainability. By embracing castor oil as a medium, artists not only enrich their work but also contribute to a more sustainable future, where creativity and environmental stewardship go hand in hand. Whether you're an artist looking to explore new techniques or simply curious about the intersection of art and sustainability, the use of castor oil presents a path worth exploring, inviting you to see the world of art through a different lens.

9.4 Castor Oil in Traditional Crafts: Reviving Old Techniques

Picture a well-worn leather satchel, its surface smooth and supple, bearing the marks of countless journeys. The secret to its enduring quality may lie in an age-old practice: conditioning with castor oil. Historically, artisans have used castor oil for leather preservation, recognizing its ability to penetrate deeply and restore flexibility. This technique, rooted in both practicality and tradition, has been a cornerstone in maintaining the longevity of leather goods. The oil's rich, viscous nature allows it to saturate the leather fibers, preventing cracking and brittleness. This process not only enhances the item's durability but also enriches its appearance, giving leather goods a timeless allure.

In candle making, castor oil has played a pivotal role in crafting candles that burn brightly and cleanly. In past centuries, communities relied on natural resources to produce light, and castor oil, with its steady burn and minimal smoke, was a preferred choice. By combining castor oil with other natural waxes, artisans created candles celebrated for their clarity and low soot production. This blend not only provided illumination but also carried cultural significance, often being used in rituals and ceremonies. The gentle flicker of a castor oil candle offered warmth and light, symbolizing hope and continuity in communal gatherings.

Today, these traditional crafts are experiencing a renaissance, as modern artisans seek to blend historical techniques with contemporary materials. The resurgence of interest in sustainable practices has encouraged crafters to revisit these methods, integrating castor oil with innovative materials to create eco-friendly products. For instance, combining castor oil with plant-based dyes and biodegradable waxes has resulted in candles that honor their historical roots while meeting today's environmental standards. This fusion of old and new not only preserves the craft but also adapts it to the current demand for sustainable and ethical goods.

Leather artisans, too, are exploring the potential of castor oil in conjunction with modern treatments. By incorporating the oil into advanced leather care products, they enhance the leather's resilience against water and environmental damage. This practice upholds the tradition of leather conditioning while providing a solution that appeals to contemporary aesthetics and functionality. The revival of these techniques speaks to a broader movement within the craft community, one that values tradition as a foundation for innovation and sustainability.

For those eager to try these crafts at home, creating natural castor oil candles is a rewarding endeavor.

- Begin by melting a blend of soy wax and beeswax in a double boiler, adding a small amount of castor oil to the mixture.

The oil's properties ensure a smooth blend that enhances the candle's burn quality.

- Once melted, pour the mixture into a mold, securing a cotton wick at the center.

- Allow it to cool and set, and you'll have a candle that not only illuminates your space but also connects you to a rich history of craftsmanship.

Conditioning leather goods with castor oil is equally straightforward.

- Start by cleaning the leather with a damp cloth to remove any surface dirt.

- Apply a small amount of castor oil to a soft cloth, and gently massage it into the leather in circular motions.

- Allow the oil to absorb overnight, then buff the surface with a clean cloth to remove any excess. This simple process will revitalize the leather, enhancing its natural luster and extending its life.

The cultural significance of these crafts is deeply rooted in the traditions of indigenous and rural communities. For generations, these techniques have been passed down, preserving the knowledge and skills that connect people to their heritage. Today, cultural preservation efforts and educational programs aim to keep these crafts alive, offering workshops and resources to those interested in learning and practicing these skills. By engaging with these traditional crafts, individuals not only develop practical skills but also contribute to the preservation of cultural heritage, ensuring that these valuable practices continue to inspire future generations.

The revival of castor oil in traditional crafts highlights a broader trend of returning to nature's gifts for sustainable living. It underscores the importance of bridging past and present, using time-honored techniques to craft items that are both functional and environmentally conscious. As you explore the possibilities of castor oil in your own creative projects, you'll find a deeper connection to the craftsmanship of the past and a path to innovate for the future.

In the next chapter, we'll explore the personal stories and expert insights that illuminate the transformative power of castor oil in everyday life. From individual testimonies of health and wellness to professional endorsements that validate its efficacy, these narratives offer a comprehensive view of how castor oil continues to impact lives around the world.

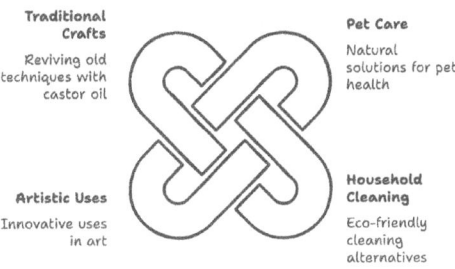

Chapter 10
Personal Stories and Expert Insights

In the quiet of evening, a mother sits at her kitchen table, the warm glow of a lamp casting comforting shadows as she gently massages castor oil onto her child's irritated skin. Her son, plagued by persistent eczema, had long struggled with discomfort and sleepless nights. Desperate for relief, she turned to castor oil after hearing about its soothing properties. Over time, she witnessed a transformation. The red, inflamed patches began to soften, and the relentless itch faded. With each application, she found hope, and her son, once restless and irritable, discovered comfort and peace (SOURCE 1). This journey highlights the powerful impact of castor oil in addressing skin conditions, offering a natural alternative that aligns with parental instincts to nurture and protect.

Across town, a senior citizen rises from his chair, the familiar creak of his knees now a distant memory. For years, he battled joint pain, an unwelcome companion that shadowed his every step. Introduced to castor oil by a friend, he was skeptical at first but decided to give it a try. He started with gentle, warm massages, applying the oil to his aching knees each evening (SOURCE 3). The change was gradual but undeniable; the stiffness eased, mobility improved, and with it, a renewed sense of independence. This experience speaks to the potential of castor oil in enhancing quality of life for those facing age-related discomfort, providing not just physical relief but emotional upliftment.

Athletes, too, have found solace in castor oil's embrace. After intense training sessions, muscles sore and fatigued, they turn to this natural remedy to aid recovery. The oil's anti-inflammatory properties help reduce swelling and promote healing, allowing them to return to their passions with vigor. Meanwhile, beauty enthusiasts revel in the glow that castor oil brings to their skincare routines. From nourishing dry skin to enhancing the health of hair and nails, its versatility is celebrated. These stories span demographics, illustrating the breadth of castor oil's applications and its ability to meet diverse needs with grace and efficacy.

The emotional and psychological impacts of such transformations are profound. When a teenager sees acne-prone skin clear, self-esteem blossoms. Confidence grows as they face the world with renewed assurance. Similarly, a woman struggling with hair loss discovers the joy of running fingers through thick, healthy locks once again, her reflection a testament to resilience and care. Castor oil, in these cases, becomes more than a treatment; it is an ally in personal journeys toward self-acceptance and empowerment.

For many, stress is a silent adversary, lurking in the shadows of daily life. Aromatherapy with castor oil offers a gentle reprieve. Infused with calming scents like lavender or chamomile, it becomes a tool for relaxation and mental clarity. Such practices remind us to pause, breathe, and find tranquility amid chaos. These anecdotes resonate deeply, for they touch on universal challenges—skin woes, aging, athletic endeavors, beauty quests, and the ever-present specter of stress.

Through the lens of personal experience, castor oil emerges as a versatile companion, ready to support and uplift, no matter the journey you find yourself on.

Reflection Section: Personal Experience Journaling

Consider keeping a journal to document your own experiences with castor oil. Note any changes in your health, beauty, or well-being. Reflect on emotional shifts and newfound confidence. This practice can offer insights and help you track progress, enhancing your journey with this natural elixir.

10.1 Expert Interviews: Insights from Natural Health Practitioners

When I sat down with Dr. Sarah Collins, an integrative medicine practitioner, her enthusiasm for castor oil was contagious. She spoke with conviction about its potential as a natural remedy, particularly its ability to enhance lymphatic drainage. "The lymphatic system is crucial for detoxification and immune function," she explained, emphasizing how castor oil massages can stimulate this often-overlooked system. Dr. Collins recommends a simple technique: Apply warmed castor oil in circular motions towards the heart, which encourages lymphatic flow and promotes overall wellness. Her insights align with a broader shift towards natural therapies that support the body's inherent healing processes.

Naturopath Dr. Evan Michaels provided further depth on castor oil's applications, particularly in holistic health. He described its anti-inflammatory properties, noting how they can be leveraged in everyday wellness routines. Dr. Michaels suggested combining castor oil with essential oils like eucalyptus for targeted muscle relief, a technique he frequently recommends to athletes seeking natural recovery options. His holistic approach paints a picture of castor oil as a versatile tool in managing both acute and chronic conditions. By integrating it into daily practices, he believes individuals can enhance their resilience and vitality.

The potential for castor oil extends beyond traditional uses. Dermatologist Dr. Lena Ramirez shared her observations on its benefits for skincare. "Castor oil is a fantastic moisturizer," she stated, highlighting its ability to penetrate deeply and nourish the skin. Dr. Ramirez often recommends it to patients with dry or sensitive skin, noting its gentle yet effective nature. Her endorsement adds credibility to the myriad anecdotal reports of castor oil's skincare benefits. Furthermore, she foresees a future where castor oil features prominently in formulations aimed at reducing the appearance of fine lines and promoting a youthful complexion.

These experts' perspectives offer a glimpse into castor oil's diverse applications and underscore its growing importance in natural health circles. Their insights validate its efficacy and encourage its broader adoption. Whether through lymphatic massages, muscle relief blends, or skincare routines, castor oil's potential continues to unfold. The expert endorsements and predictions not only reinforce its current uses but also hint at exciting possibilities for future applications.

10.2 Testimonials: Real-Life Benefits and Experiences

Imagine gathering around a table, a diverse group of individuals sharing stories of transformation, each voice unique but united by a common thread—castor oil. Among them, eco-conscious consumers speak of their commitment to sustainable living. They have embraced castor oil not just for its benefits, but for its alignment with environmental values. One young woman shares how she replaced chemical-laden hair products with castor oil, experiencing not only enhanced hair health but also a lighter ecological footprint. Her journey mirrors that of many who seek harmony between personal care and planet care, finding in castor oil a partner in both beauty and sustainability.

Holistic health advocates, familiar with natural remedies, often find castor oil a staple in their wellness routines. They recount stories of improved digestion and detoxification, describing how regular use of castor oil packs has revitalized their systems. One advocate mentions a newfound energy after incorporating castor oil into her cleansing rituals, attributing her vitality to its detoxifying properties. These experiences highlight the tangible health benefits that extend beyond the surface, offering deeper connections to bodily rhythms and natural cycles. With each testimonial, the narrative of castor oil as a holistic health enhancer grows richer, resonating with those seeking authentic, natural solutions.

Skeptics often approach natural remedies with caution, yet many find their doubts dispelled through firsthand experience. A father, initially wary of natural solutions, shares how castor oil addressed his persistent digestive issues. His skepticism gave way to belief as he witnessed real, lasting improvements. These accounts address common hesitations, showing how castor oil bridges the gap between doubt and acceptance. By sharing their experiences, these individuals offer encouragement to others who may be hesitant, illustrating that trust in natural remedies can yield profound results.

The authenticity of these stories lies in their relatability. They reflect the everyday struggles and triumphs of people from all walks of life. Anecdotes about healthier hair, better digestion, and eco-friendly choices echo challenges faced by many, providing a mirror for readers. This genuine storytelling fosters connection, drawing you into a community where castor oil is not just a product but a catalyst for positive change. Through these voices, the transformative power of castor oil becomes vividly clear, inviting you to consider its place in your own life.

10.3 Insider Tips: Maximizing Castor Oil Benefits

Incorporating castor oil into your daily routine can be as simple as adding a few drops to your favorite moisturizer or shampoo. For skin, apply a small amount to damp skin to lock in moisture. This method helps prevent that oily residue which can occur if too much product is used. For hair, mix it with lighter oils like jojoba or argan to create a nourishing treatment that won't weigh down your locks. Applying a warm towel after application can enhance absorption by opening up your pores or hair cuticles, allowing the oil to penetrate more deeply and effectively.

Avoid common mistakes such as overuse, which often leads to an oily build-up that can clog pores or leave hair greasy. More isn't always better, so start with a small amount and adjust as needed. When crafting DIY projects, remember that castor oil can be a versatile ingredient beyond beauty. It can be combined with other natural elements to create household polishes and cleaners. Mix it with lemon juice and vinegar for a homemade furniture polish or with baking soda for a gentle scrub. These projects not only offer practical uses but also reduce reliance on chemical-laden products.

When creating personalized blends, consider the specific needs you wish to address. Adding essential oils can target particular concerns. Lavender essential oil can enhance relaxation when used in massages, while tea tree oil adds an antimicrobial boost for acne-prone skin. For a refreshing scent, citrus oils like lemon or orange can invigorate and uplift. Customizing your blend allows you to tailor the benefits of castor oil to your unique preferences and needs, expanding its application from a simple oil to a key component in your personalized wellness toolkit.

10.4 The Future of Castor Oil: Trends and Innovations

Castor oil, a staple in traditional medicine, is now stepping onto a broader stage in the modern world. One of the most exciting developments is its role in sustainable fashion and textiles. Designers and manufacturers are increasingly turning to castor oil for its eco-friendly properties. It is used in dyeing processes that enhance color absorption and provide water resistance, making it ideal for outdoor clothing. Additionally, castor oil-based fibers are gaining traction, offering a renewable alternative to synthetic materials. This shift not only reflects a growing consumer demand for sustainable products but also highlights the versatility of castor oil beyond traditional uses.

In technology, castor oil extraction and refinement have seen remarkable advancements. The cold-pressed method, which preserves the oil's natural properties, has been refined to increase efficiency and reduce waste. Innovations in machinery have made it possible to extract oil with minimal environmental impact, aligning with eco-friendly packaging solutions. Companies are now exploring biodegradable packaging made from castor oil derivatives, reducing the reliance on plastics. These developments are part of a broader movement towards sustainability, where castor oil plays a pivotal role in reducing ecological footprints.

Looking ahead, market trends suggest a surge in demand for organic and ethically sourced oils. Consumers are becoming more conscious of the origins of their products, seeking assurances of purity and sustainability. This shift is likely to drive the castor oil industry towards more transparent and ethical practices. Additionally, research and development continue to unlock new potential. Clinical trials are underway to explore castor oil's health benefits, with promising results in areas such as anti-inflammatory and antimicrobial applications. There's also significant interest in developing pharmaceuticals based on castor oil, offering natural alternatives to conventional medications.

The future of castor oil is bright, with innovations spanning multiple industries. As research progresses, we can expect breakthroughs that will further cement castor oil's place in both health and environmental solutions. The ongoing exploration into its applications promises not only to enhance our understanding but also to expand the possibilities for its use, shaping the way we approach sustainability and wellness.

10.5 Interactive Experience: Enhancing Learning with QR Codes

In today's digital age, merging traditional reading with interactive elements can significantly enrich your learning experience. Imagine flipping through these pages and pausing to scan a QR code that leads you to an engaging video demonstration. Suddenly, the text you're reading about using castor oil for skin care comes alive with a step-by-step visual guide. This approach caters to visual learners who benefit from seeing processes in action. QR codes offer access to a wealth of information beyond the printed page, connecting you to expert interviews where practitioners share their insights on castor oil's varied applications, or to detailed studies that delve into its scientific underpinnings. This integration of digital content transforms the book into a dynamic resource, adapting to different learning styles and preferences. By bridging the gap between static text and interactive media, QR codes invite you to explore and understand castor oil's benefits in a more comprehensive way.

With each scan, you'll find new pathways to deepen your understanding. A QR code beside a recipe for a castor oil hair mask might lead you to a video tutorial, showing exactly how to mix and apply the ingredients for optimal results. Another code might transport you to an expert panel discussion, offering diverse perspectives on castor oil's role in holistic wellness. This interactive layer not only enhances comprehension but also keeps the learning process engaging and immersive. By providing multiple avenues to explore, QR codes ensure that the content is accessible to everyone, whether you prefer reading, watching, or listening.

Moreover, this approach fosters a sense of community and collaboration. As you interact with these digital elements, you're encouraged to share your experiences and insights through online platforms. These forums become a space to exchange tips, discuss outcomes, and support one another in your castor oil journey. Sharing stories and feedback creates a network of like-minded individuals, all learning and growing together. This collective wisdom not only enriches your own knowledge but also contributes to a broader understanding of castor oil's potential. By embracing this interactive experience, you become an active participant in a vibrant, evolving dialogue about natural health and wellness.

10.6 Beyond Borders: Castor Oil's Global Impact

Across the vibrant landscapes of South America, castor oil has been a cornerstone in traditional healing practices for generations. Communities utilize it not just for its medicinal properties but also for its role in daily life. In Brazil, for instance, it is often used to soothe skin ailments and as a natural remedy for digestive issues. These uses are deeply rooted in cultural traditions, where knowledge is passed down through generations, maintaining a connection to the earth and its natural resources. This relationship with castor oil underscores a broader respect for nature's ability to heal and sustain.

In Europe, the allure of castor oil has been rekindled in the beauty industry, where its rich properties are celebrated in modern skincare routines. From high-end boutiques in Paris to quaint apothecaries in London, castor oil is a favored ingredient for its moisturizing and rejuvenating qualities. It is often found in serums and creams, touted for its ability to enhance skin elasticity and promote a youthful glow. This modern adaptation highlights the versatile nature of castor oil, proving that ancient remedies can find new life in contemporary settings, bridging the past with the present in a seamless blend of tradition and innovation.

The global market for castor oil is a dynamic landscape, driven by both demand and heritage. Major exporting countries like India and Brazil dominate the market, providing a substantial share of the world's supply. These nations leverage their rich agricultural resources and expertise in castor cultivation to meet the growing demand. This trade is not just about economics; it is a cultural exchange that allows different regions to share their unique uses and applications. As countries trade castor oil, they also exchange knowledge, techniques, and innovations, enriching the global understanding of this remarkable oil.

Throughout history, castor oil has facilitated cultural exchange and adaptation. The influence of Ayurvedic practices, for example, has permeated Western wellness trends, bringing holistic approaches to health into mainstream consciousness. As Western societies embrace these practices, they adapt and integrate them, creating a fusion of philosophies that enriches both cultures. This cross-pollination of ideas is a testament to castor oil's universal appeal, transcending geographical boundaries to become a symbol of shared knowledge and mutual respect. It is not merely a product but a catalyst for connection, bridging diverse cultures through a common appreciation for its versatile benefits.

10.7 Your Wellness Journey: Embracing Castor Oil for Life

Incorporating castor oil into your wellness routine can be a transformative step towards holistic health. As you embark on this path, consider setting clear personal health goals that align with your needs and aspirations. Whether it's improving your skin's texture, enhancing hair growth, or supporting your immune system, clearly defined goals can provide direction and motivation. Begin by assessing your current health status and identify areas where castor oil could be beneficial. This might involve a simple evening ritual of applying it to your skin, or a weekly hair treatment to restore shine and vitality. By integrating castor oil into your life with purpose, you're not just using a product; you're embracing a natural lifestyle.

The long-term benefits of regular castor oil use are profound. Consistent application can lead to sustained improvements in both skin and hair health. Its moisturizing properties help maintain elasticity and prevent dryness, while its nourishing components support hair strength and luster. Beyond aesthetics, castor oil plays a significant role in immune support. Its ability to enhance lymphatic function can contribute to a healthier immune system, keeping you resilient against seasonal challenges. Over time, these benefits accumulate, reflecting a commitment to self-care that extends beyond mere surface-level beauty. This continuity in practice nurtures a robust foundation for overall well-being.

To effectively incorporate castor oil into your personal wellness plan, consider creating a structured framework. Journaling can be a valuable tool, allowing you to track the changes and improvements you experience. Document your journey with a simple template that includes sections for noting weekly goals, daily observations, and any adjustments you make along the way. This practice provides clarity and insight, helping you understand how your body responds to castor oil. Be open to adapting your routine as life changes, whether it's due to seasonal shifts, lifestyle adjustments, or evolving health needs. Flexibility is key to maintaining a routine that serves you effectively.

Sustainability and mindfulness are integral to this approach. As you use castor oil, reflect on its origins and the environmental impact of your choices. Engage in this practice with gratitude, acknowledging the natural resources that make it possible. This mindset fosters a deeper connection to the earth and encourages sustainable practices that benefit both you and the planet. By cultivating mindfulness, each application of castor oil becomes an opportunity to center yourself, promote balance, and express gratitude for the simple, natural solutions that enhance your life.

In this chapter, we've explored integrating castor oil into personal wellness routines, emphasizing the importance of setting goals and tracking progress. As you move forward, consider how this aligns with broader health practices.

Conclusion

As we reach the end of our journey through the rich and multifaceted world of castor oil, let's take a moment to reflect on the insights and knowledge we've uncovered together. From its ancient roots in civilizations such as Egypt and India to its modern-day applications, castor oil has proven itself to be a powerful ally in health, beauty, and sustainable living. We've explored its scientifically supported benefits, from reducing inflammation and enhancing skin health to boosting immunity and promoting hair growth. Throughout these pages, personal stories and expert insights have brought these benefits to life, offering real-world examples of castor oil's transformative power.

One of the key takeaways from our exploration is the importance of authenticity. Identifying pure castor oil and understanding how to use it effectively can unlock a world of benefits. Whether it's through soothing skin conditions, nourishing hair, or enhancing your wellness routine, the versatility of castor oil is truly remarkable. By incorporating it into your daily life, you can embrace a more holistic approach to health, one that aligns with the rhythms of nature and supports your body's natural healing processes.

I encourage you to continue experimenting with the recipes, techniques, and rituals we've shared. Let castor oil be a tool for creativity and personalization in your wellness journey. Try different combina-

THE HIDDEN POWER OF CASTOR OIL: NATURE'S... 113

tions, adapt them to your needs, and discover what works best for you. Share your experiences with friends and family and invite them to join you on this path of natural health exploration. The beauty of castor oil lies in its adaptability, allowing each person to tailor its use to their unique preferences and lifestyle.

Beyond personal health, embracing castor oil is a step towards sustainable and mindful living. Each choice you make has an impact, and by opting for eco-friendly products like castor oil, you're contributing to a healthier planet. Consider the environmental footprint of your lifestyle decisions and choose options that support a sustainable future. Every small action counts, and together, we can make a significant difference.

As you integrate the principles and practices discussed in this book into your broader wellness journey, I hope you'll embrace a holistic lifestyle. This approach goes beyond castor oil, encompassing other natural and sustainable practices that nurture both body and soul. By doing so, you cultivate a balanced life that's in harmony with nature, fostering well-being in every aspect.

I want to express my heartfelt gratitude for joining me on this journey. My passion for natural remedies and helping others achieve balanced, healthy lifestyles is what drives me. I'm committed to providing trustworthy, simple guidance that empowers you to make informed decisions about your health and well-being.

It's been a privilege to share these ancient holistic secrets with you and empower you to embrace natural, chemical-free approaches to health and wellness.

Your feedback and experiences are invaluable. I invite you to share your thoughts, with others by leaving a review on Amazon. Your feedback not only helps others make informed decisions but also spreads the message of natural, holistic living.

To leave a review, visit the book's page on Amazon, simply use the QR Code below to take you to the relevant page.

Whether it's a short note about your favourite tip or how you've begun using castor oil, every review makes a difference.

A Note From The Author

Dear Reader,

As we close, remember this: "Nature itself is the best physician." Let this thought guide you as you continue to explore the wonders of castor oil and beyond. May your journey towards health, wellness, and sustainability be filled with discovery and joy. With castor oil as your trusted companion, the possibilities are endless.

Your feedback and experiences are invaluable. I invite you to share your thoughts, with others by leaving a review on Amazon. Your feedback not only helps others make informed decisions but also spreads the message of natural, holistic living.

To leave a review, visit the book's page on Amazon, simply use the QR Code below to take you to the relevant page.

Whether it's a short note about your favourite tip or how you've begun using castor oil, every review makes a difference. Thank you for supporting this mission of sharing nature's powerful remedies with the world!

Together, we can learn, grow, and inspire each other.
Thank you for allowing me to be a part of your journey.
Barbara Harris

The Hidden Power Of Castor Oil

Nature's Ultimate Elixir: Bonus Recipes

HEALTH & WELLNESS USES
DIGESTIVE HEALTH
1. Classic Castor Oil Digestive Cleanse

A gentle overnight remedy for occasional constipation

Ingredients:

- 1-2 teaspoons of cold-pressed, hexane-free castor oil

- 1 tablespoon of fresh orange juice or warm ginger tea (optional, to improve taste)

Directions:

1. Measure castor oil into a small spoon.

2. If desired, mix with orange juice or take followed by warm

ginger tea to mask the taste.

3. Take on an empty stomach before bedtime.

4. Expect results within 6-8 hours.

Usage Notes:
- Not recommended for regular use; limit to occasional relief
- Not suitable during pregnancy or menstruation
- Discontinue if cramping becomes uncomfortable

2. Digestive Massage Oil Blend

A gentle abdominal massage to support digestive movement

Ingredients:
- 2 tablespoons castor oil
- 5 drops ginger essential oil
- 3 drops peppermint essential oil
- Small glass bowl
- Hot water bottle or heating pad

Directions:

1. Mix oils in a small glass bowl.

2. Warm the mixture by placing the bowl in hot water for 2 minutes.

3. Apply to abdomen in clockwise circular motions for 10-15 minutes.

4. Cover with a thin cotton cloth and apply heat with a hot water bottle.

5. Rest for 30-45 minutes.

Usage Notes:
- Best done 1-2 times weekly
- Avoid during active digestive upset
- Store remaining oil in a dark glass bottle

JOINT & MUSCLE RELIEF

1. Warming Castor Oil Joint Rub

Deep-penetrating relief for arthritic joints and stiffness

Ingredients:

- 3 tablespoons castor oil
- 10 drops eucalyptus essential oil
- 7 drops rosemary essential oil
- 5 drops ginger essential oil
- Dark glass bottle for storage

Directions:

1. Combine all oils in a dark glass bottle and shake well.
2. Warm a small amount between palms.
3. Massage into affected joints using firm, circular motions.
4. Cover with a warm compress or wrap with a wool scarf.
5. Leave on for 30-60 minutes or overnight.

Usage Notes:

- Apply 1-3 times daily as needed
- Patch test first for sensitivity
- Can stain fabrics; use old clothes/towels

2. Anti-Inflammatory Cold Compress

For acute inflammation and swelling

Ingredients:

- ¼ cup castor oil
- 8 drops peppermint essential oil
- Cotton flannel cloth
- Plastic wrap
- Small towel
- Ice pack

Directions:

1. Mix castor oil with peppermint essential oil.
2. Fold flannel cloth and soak in the oil mixture.
3. Apply to affected area.
4. Cover with plastic wrap, then place ice pack over the area.
5. Secure with towel and leave for 20 minutes.

Usage Notes:

- Best for recent injuries with inflammation
- Allow 2-3 hours between applications
- Not for use on broken skin

3. Castor Oil Runner's Relief Bath

Post-exercise muscle recovery soak

Ingredients:

- 3 tablespoons castor oil
- 1 cup Epsom salts
- 10 drops lavender essential oil
- 5 drops marjoram essential oil
- Warm bath water

Directions:
1. Fill tub with warm water.
2. Mix castor oil with essential oils in a small bowl.
3. Add this mixture and Epsom salts to the bath.
4. Stir water to disperse oils.
5. Soak for 20-30 minutes.

Usage Notes:
- Use caution entering and exiting tub as surfaces may be slippery
- Hydrate well after bath
- Limit to once weekly

IMMUNE SYSTEM BOOST

1. Classic Castor Oil Pack for Lymphatic Support

Traditional method to support lymphatic drainage

Ingredients:

- ½ cup organic, cold-pressed castor oil
- 100% cotton or wool flannel cloth (approximately 12" x 14")
- Hot water bottle or heating pad
- Old towel
- Plastic wrap
- Storage container for the cloth

Directions:

1. Fold flannel into a rectangle that covers desired area.
2. Pour castor oil onto cloth until saturated but not dripping.
3. Apply cloth over abdomen, covering liver area (right side under ribs).
4. Cover with plastic wrap, then place heating pad on top.
5. Wrap with old towel to secure.
6. Rest for 45-60 minutes.
7. Store cloth in container for future use (can be reused 25-30 times).

Usage Notes:

- Best done 3-4 times weekly for lymphatic support

- Avoid during menstruation or pregnancy
- May induce detoxification symptoms; start slowly

2. Immune-Boosting Chest Rub

Supportive care during seasonal transitions

Ingredients:
- 2 tablespoons castor oil
- 4 drops eucalyptus essential oil
- 3 drops tea tree essential oil
- 3 drops thyme essential oil
- Small glass jar

Directions:
1. Combine all ingredients in glass jar and mix well.
2. Apply a thin layer to chest, throat, and upper back.
3. Cover with a warm, dry cloth.
4. Rest for 20-30 minutes.
5. Can be left on overnight.

Usage Notes:
- Use at first sign of seasonal discomfort
- Not recommended for children under 12
- Store in cool, dark place for up to 3 months

HORMONAL BALANCE

1. Hormone-Balancing Abdominal Pack

Traditional approach for menstrual discomfort and hormonal support

Ingredients:

- ⅓ cup castor oil
- 100% wool or cotton flannel cloth
- Hot water bottle or heating pad
- Old towel or wrap
- Plastic wrap

Directions:

1. Fold flannel to fit lower abdomen.
2. Saturate cloth with castor oil.
3. Apply to lower abdomen, covering from navel to pubic bone.
4. Cover with plastic wrap.
5. Place heating pad over pack.
6. Secure with towel or wrap.
7. Rest for 30-60 minutes.
8. Store cloth in container for future use.

Usage Notes:

- Best used 3 times weekly between menstrual periods

- Discontinue during active menstruation
- Not for use during pregnancy
- May initially intensify symptoms before improvement

2. PMS Support Massage Oil

For targeted relief of premenstrual discomfort

Ingredients:

- 2 tablespoons castor oil
- 1 tablespoon evening primrose oil
- 5 drops clary sage essential oil
- 3 drops lavender essential oil
- Dark glass bottle

Directions:

1. Combine all oils in dark glass bottle.
2. Shake well before each use.
3. Warm 1-2 teaspoons between palms.
4. Massage into lower abdomen using gentle, clockwise motions.
5. Apply warm compress after massage.
6. Rest for 15-20 minutes.

Usage Notes:

- Begin 7-10 days before expected period
- Discontinue during menstruation
- Not for use during pregnancy
- Store in cool, dark place

LIVER DETOX

1. Traditional Liver Support Castor Oil Pack

Classic method for liver detoxification support

Ingredients:

- ½ cup organic, cold-pressed castor oil
- 100% wool flannel cloth (approximately 12" x 14")
- Hot water bottle or heating pad
- Old towel
- Plastic wrap
- Glass container with lid for storage

Directions:

1. Fold flannel to fit over liver area (right side under ribcage).
2. Pour castor oil onto cloth until saturated but not dripping.
3. Apply cloth directly over liver area.
4. Cover with plastic wrap.
5. Place heating pad over pack and secure with old towel.
6. Rest for 45-60 minutes.
7. Store cloth in glass container (can be reused 25-30 times).

Usage Notes:

- Best done 3-4 times weekly for 4-6 weeks
- Avoid during illness, menstruation, or pregnancy

- May trigger detoxification reactions; start with shorter sessions

- Support with increased water intake

2. Morning Liver Flush

Gentle morning support for liver function

Ingredients:

- ½ teaspoon castor oil
- Juice of ½ lemon
- 1 cup warm water
- ¼ teaspoon turmeric powder
- Pinch of black pepper
- 1 teaspoon raw honey (optional)

Directions:

1. Heat water until warm but not boiling.
2. Add all ingredients and stir well.
3. Drink on an empty stomach first thing in the morning.

Usage Notes:

- Start with once weekly, gradually increasing to 2-3 times weekly
- Not recommended for daily use
- Discontinue if digestive discomfort occurs

- Not suitable during pregnancy

SKIN & BEAUTY
DEEP MOISTURIZER

1. Overnight Intensive Moisture Treatment

Deep hydration for extremely dry skin

Ingredients:
- 1 tablespoon castor oil
- 2 teaspoons jojoba or sweet almond oil
- 3 drops lavender essential oil (optional)
- Cotton gloves and socks (for hands and feet)

Directions:
1. Mix all oils in a small bowl.
2. After evening cleansing, apply a thin layer to clean, slightly damp skin.
3. For hands and feet, apply generously then cover with cotton gloves/socks.
4. Leave overnight.
5. Rinse with warm water in the morning.

Usage Notes:
- Use 2-3 times weekly for dry skin
- For facial use, apply very sparingly to avoid clogging pores
- Patch test first, especially for sensitive skin

2. Nourishing Lip Treatment

Intensive repair for chapped or dry lips

Ingredients:

- ½ teaspoon castor oil
- ½ teaspoon honey
- ¼ teaspoon vitamin E oil
- Small container for storage

Directions:

1. Mix all ingredients thoroughly.
2. Apply to clean lips with fingertip.
3. Leave on for at least 30 minutes or overnight.
4. For daytime, blot excess with tissue before applying makeup.

Usage Notes:

- Can be used daily
- Store in cool, dark place for up to 2 weeks
- Avoid if allergic to bee products

3. Cuticle & Nail Strengthening Oil

Nourishing treatment for brittle nails and dry cuticles

Ingredients:

- 1 tablespoon castor oil
- 1 teaspoon olive oil

- 5 drops lemon essential oil
- Small dropper bottle

Directions:
1. Combine all oils in dropper bottle.
2. Shake well before use.
3. Apply 1-2 drops to each cuticle.
4. Massage into nails and surrounding skin.
5. Best applied before bed.

Usage Notes:
- Use daily for best results
- Can be used before manicures to soften cuticles
- Avoid if you have citrus allergies

WRINKLE & FINE LINE REDUCTION

1. Anti-Aging Night Serum

Nourishing facial treatment to minimize fine lines

Ingredients:
- 1 teaspoon castor oil
- 2 teaspoons rosehip seed oil
- 3 drops frankincense essential oil
- 2 drops lavender essential oil
- Dark glass dropper bottle

Directions:
1. Combine all oils in dropper bottle.
2. Shake gently before each use.
3. After cleansing and toning, apply 3-4 drops to slightly damp skin.
4. Gently massage using upward motions.
5. Allow to absorb for 10 minutes before lying down.

Usage Notes:
- Use every other night
- Adjust amount based on skin's absorption
- Discontinue if any irritation occurs
- Store in cool, dark place for up to 3 months

2. Expression Line Smoothing Oil

Targeted treatment for forehead and eye area

Ingredients:

- ½ teaspoon castor oil
- ½ teaspoon argan oil
- 3 drops carrot seed essential oil
- Small glass jar

Directions:

1. Mix oils thoroughly in glass jar.
2. After evening cleansing, dab a tiny amount onto fingertip.
3. Apply with light tapping motions to forehead lines, crow's feet, and between brows.
4. Allow to absorb overnight.

Usage Notes:

- Use 3-4 times weekly
- Avoid getting in eyes
- Use very sparingly—a little goes a long way
- May increase sun sensitivity; use sunscreen during the day

ACNE TREATMENT

1. Clarifying Castor Oil Spot Treatment

Targeted overnight treatment for individual blemishes

Ingredients:

- 1 teaspoon castor oil
- 2 drops tea tree essential oil
- 1 drop lavender essential oil
- Small glass jar

Directions:

1. Mix oils thoroughly in glass jar.
2. Cleanse face and apply regular skincare.
3. Dip a clean cotton swab into the mixture.
4. Apply directly to blemishes, avoiding surrounding skin.
5. Leave overnight.
6. Rinse thoroughly in the morning.

Usage Notes:

- Use only as a spot treatment
- Discontinue if irritation occurs
- Not recommended for cystic acne
- Store in cool, dark place for up to 1 month

2. Purifying Clay & Castor Oil Mask

Weekly treatment to draw out impurities and balance oil production

Ingredients:

- 1 tablespoon bentonite or kaolin clay
- 1 teaspoon castor oil
- 1 teaspoon raw honey
- 3-5 drops tea tree essential oil
- Enough filtered water to create a paste

Directions:

1. Mix clay, castor oil, and honey in a non-metal bowl.
2. Add essential oil and enough water to form a smooth paste.
3. Apply to clean skin, avoiding eye area.
4. Allow to dry for 10-15 minutes (should not completely harden).
5. Rinse with warm water using gentle circular motions.
6. Follow with moisturizer.

Usage Notes:

- Use once weekly for oily/acne-prone skin
- Prepare fresh for each use
- May cause temporary redness that should subside within 30 minutes

- Not recommended for very dry or sensitive skin

SCAR & STRETCH MARK REDUCTION
1. Regenerative Scar Treatment Oil
Consistent care to improve scar appearance

Ingredients:
- 1 tablespoon castor oil
- 1 tablespoon rosehip seed oil
- 5 drops helichrysum essential oil
- 5 drops frankincense essential oil
- Dark glass bottle with dropper

Directions:
1. Combine all oils in bottle and mix well.
2. Cleanse affected area.
3. Apply 5-10 drops (depending on area size) to scar tissue.
4. Massage using circular motions for 3-5 minutes to increase circulation.
5. Apply twice daily for best results.

Usage Notes:
- Consistency is key—use regularly for at least 8-12 weeks
- Safe for old scars, but wait until new scars are fully closed
- Avoid on broken skin
- May stain clothing; allow to absorb before dressing

2. Pregnancy Stretch Mark Prevention Blend

Moisturizing oil to support skin elasticity during pregnancy

Ingredients:
- 2 tablespoons castor oil
- 2 tablespoons sweet almond oil
- 1 tablespoon cocoa butter, melted
- 5 drops lavender essential oil
- 3 drops neroli essential oil (optional)
- Glass jar with tight-fitting lid

Directions:
1. Melt cocoa butter using a double boiler.
2. Remove from heat and add all other ingredients.
3. Pour into glass jar and allow to cool.
4. Apply to clean skin on abdomen, hips, thighs, and breasts twice daily.
5. Massage into skin using circular motions until absorbed.

Usage Notes:
- Begin in first trimester and continue postpartum
- Perform patch test before full application
- Avoid essential oils if sensitive or if advised by healthcare provider

- Store at room temperature for up to 3 months

DARK CIRCLE & PUFFY EYE TREATMENT
1. Overnight Eye Rejuvenation Treatment
Gentle care for under-eye circles and puffiness

Ingredients:

- ½ teaspoon castor oil
- ½ teaspoon rosehip seed oil
- 1 drop chamomile essential oil (optional)
- Small glass jar

Directions:

1. Mix oils thoroughly in glass jar.
2. Before bed, wash face and apply regular skincare.
3. Dip clean ring finger into oil mixture.
4. Gently pat a tiny amount along orbital bone (not on lids or too close to eyes).
5. Leave overnight.
6. Rinse in morning.

Usage Notes:

- Use very sparingly—a few drops is sufficient
- Keep away from lash line and tear ducts
- Discontinue if any irritation occurs
- Store in cool, dark place

2. Cooling Eye De-Puffer

Quick morning remedy for puffy eyes

Ingredients:
- 1 teaspoon castor oil
- 2 stainless steel spoons
- Small bowl of ice water

Directions:
1. Place spoons in ice water for 5 minutes.
2. Apply a thin layer of castor oil under eyes.
3. Remove spoons from ice water and dry.
4. Place the backs of the cold spoons against puffy areas.
5. Hold for 30 seconds, then repeat 2-3 times.
6. Leave remaining oil as a treatment or blot excess with tissue.

Usage Notes:
- Ideal for morning use
- Can be repeated throughout day if needed
- Refrigerating castor oil enhances the cooling effect
- Use clean spoons each time

HAIR & SCALP CARE
HAIR GROWTH STIMULATOR

1. Intensive Scalp Treatment for Hair Growth

Weekly ritual to nourish follicles and encourage growth

Ingredients:

- 2 tablespoons castor oil
- 1 tablespoon coconut oil
- 5 drops rosemary essential oil
- 3 drops peppermint essential oil
- Shower cap or towel
- Wide-tooth comb

Directions:

1. Mix oils in a small bowl.
2. Warm mixture by placing bowl in hot water for 2 minutes.
3. Section dry hair and apply oil directly to scalp with fingertips.
4. Massage scalp using circular motions for 5-10 minutes.
5. Cover with shower cap or warm towel.
6. Leave for 1-2 hours or overnight.
7. Shampoo twice to remove oil completely.

Usage Notes:

- Use weekly for best results

- May need extra shampoo to fully remove

- Reduce amount for fine or thin hair

- Can stain pillowcases; use old cases if leaving overnight

2. Daily Scalp Stimulating Drops

Regular maintenance for ongoing hair health

Ingredients:

- 1 tablespoon castor oil

- 2 tablespoons aloe vera gel

- 10 drops rosemary essential oil

- 5 drops cedarwood essential oil

- Small glass dropper bottle

Directions:

1. Combine all ingredients in bottle and shake well before each use.

2. Apply 5-10 drops to scalp, focusing on thinning areas.

3. Massage in with fingertips for 3-5 minutes.

4. Leave in—no need to rinse out.

5. Apply to dry or slightly damp hair before bed or 30 minutes before styling.

Usage Notes:

- Shake well before each use as ingredients may separate

- Use daily for 3 months minimum to see results
- Will not cause oiliness when used in small amounts
- Store in refrigerator for up to 2 weeks

DANDRUFF & SCALP HEALTH

1. Clarifying Scalp Treatment

Deep treatment for flaky, itchy scalp

Ingredients:

- 3 tablespoons castor oil
- 1 tablespoon apple cider vinegar
- 5 drops tea tree essential oil
- 3 drops lavender essential oil
- Shower cap
- Small spray bottle with water (for rinsing)

Directions:

1. Mix oils and vinegar in a small bowl.
2. Apply to dry scalp in sections, focusing on problem areas.
3. Massage thoroughly for 5-10 minutes.
4. Cover with shower cap.
5. Leave for 30-60 minutes.
6. Before shampooing, spritz with water and massage again to emulsify oil.
7. Shampoo twice to remove completely.

Usage Notes:

- Use weekly until condition improves, then every 2 weeks

- Vinegar smell dissipates after rinsing
- Perform patch test first, as tea tree can be sensitizing
- May temporarily sting if scalp has scratches

2. Cooling Peppermint Scalp Tonic

Refreshing relief for itchy, irritated scalp

Ingredients:
- 1 tablespoon castor oil
- 3 tablespoons witch hazel
- 10 drops peppermint essential oil
- 5 drops rosemary essential oil
- Small spray bottle

Directions:
1. Combine all ingredients in spray bottle.
2. Shake well before each use.
3. Part hair in several places and spray directly onto scalp.
4. Massage in with fingertips.
5. No need to rinse out.
6. Can be applied to dry or damp hair.

Usage Notes:
- Use as needed for itching or irritation

- Avoid if you have very dry hair, as witch hazel can be drying
- Refrigerate for enhanced cooling effect
- Store for up to 3 weeks

EYEBROW & EYELASH GROWTH
1. Overnight Lash & Brow Serum
Nourishing treatment for fuller lashes and brows

Ingredients:
- 1 teaspoon castor oil
- ¼ teaspoon vitamin E oil
- Clean mascara wand or small brush
- Small glass container

Directions:
1. Mix oils in glass container.
2. Remove all makeup and cleanse lash line and brows.
3. Dip clean mascara wand or brush into oil mixture.
4. Apply sparingly to clean eyebrows, brushing in direction of hair growth.
5. For lashes, apply to base of lash line (like applying eyeliner) with a cotton swab.
6. Leave overnight.
7. Rinse in morning.

Usage Notes:
- Use daily for best results
- Avoid getting oil in eyes
- Results typically seen after 6-8 weeks of consistent use

- If irritation occurs, discontinue immediately

SPLIT END REPAIR

1. Intensive Split End Mending Treatment

Temporary repair for damaged hair ends

Ingredients:
- 1 tablespoon castor oil
- 1 teaspoon argan oil
- ½ teaspoon honey
- Small glass jar

Directions:

1. Mix all ingredients thoroughly.

2. Apply to dry hair, focusing on the bottom 2-3 inches.

3. Pay special attention to visibly split or frayed ends.

4. Leave for 30 minutes to 2 hours.

5. Shampoo and condition as normal.

Usage Notes:
- Use once weekly for maintenance
- For severely damaged hair, use twice weekly
- Can be applied to damp hair before air-drying to smooth ends
- Remember this is a temporary fix; regular trims are still nec-

THE HIDDEN POWER OF CASTOR OIL: NATURE'S... 153

essary

PRE-SHAMPOO SCALP TREATMENT
1. Balancing Pre-Shampoo Oil Treatment
Deep conditioning preparation for wash day

Ingredients:

- 2 tablespoons castor oil
- 1 tablespoon jojoba oil
- 1 tablespoon olive oil
- 5 drops lavender essential oil
- Wide-tooth comb
- Shower cap

Directions:

1. Mix all oils in a bowl.
2. Section dry hair and apply oil mixture directly to scalp first.
3. Massage thoroughly for 5-10 minutes.
4. Distribute remaining oil through length of hair, focusing on ends.
5. Gently comb to ensure even distribution.
6. Cover with shower cap.
7. Leave for 30 minutes to overnight.
8. Shampoo thoroughly, possibly twice.

Usage Notes:

THE HIDDEN POWER OF CASTOR OIL: NATURE'S...

- Use before regular wash day, 1-2 times monthly
- For very dry hair and scalp, leave overnight
- For fine hair, focus primarily on scalp and ends
- May require double shampooing to remove completely

HOLISTIC & ALTERNATIVE HEALING
WOUND HEALING

1. Simple Wound Care Salve

Basic protection for minor cuts and abrasions

Ingredients:

- 1 tablespoon castor oil
- 1 tablespoon coconut oil
- 5 drops lavender essential oil
- 3 drops tea tree essential oil
- Small glass jar with lid

Directions:

1. Melt coconut oil if solid.
2. Mix all ingredients thoroughly.
3. Allow to cool and solidify slightly.
4. Clean wound gently with mild soap and water.
5. Apply a thin layer of salve with clean fingertip or cotton swab.

6. Cover with sterile bandage if needed.

7. Reapply 2-3 times daily.

Usage Notes:
- For minor cuts, scrapes, and burns only

- Do not use on deep wounds, punctures, or severely infected areas

- Discontinue if irritation occurs

- Seek medical attention for serious wounds or if infection develops

SINUS & ALLERGY RELIEF
1. Sinus Pressure Relief Massage Oil
Targeted application for congestion and pressure

Ingredients:

- 1 tablespoon castor oil
- 3 drops eucalyptus essential oil
- 2 drops peppermint essential oil
- 2 drops rosemary essential oil
- Small glass jar

Directions:

1. Mix all oils in glass jar.
2. Warm a small amount between fingertips.
3. Apply to bridge of nose, temples, forehead, and behind ears.
4. Using ring fingers, apply gentle pressure and small circular motions to sides of nose.
5. Continue massage for 3-5 minutes.
6. Leave oil on for at least 30 minutes or overnight.

Usage Notes:

- Use up to 3 times daily during congestion
- Keep away from eyes
- Not recommended for children under 10

- Discontinue if headache worsens

SLEEP & RELAXATION AID
1. Calming Foot Treatment for Better Sleep
Relaxing bedtime ritual to promote restful sleep

Ingredients:
- 1 tablespoon castor oil
- 3 drops lavender essential oil
- 2 drops chamomile essential oil
- Cotton socks
- Small basin of hot water (optional)

Directions:
1. Mix castor oil with essential oils.
2. Soak feet in hot water for 5 minutes if desired.
3. Dry feet thoroughly.
4. Apply oil mixture generously to soles of feet, focusing on pressure points.
5. Massage for 2-3 minutes.
6. Put on cotton socks.
7. Leave overnight.

Usage Notes:
- Use 30-60 minutes before bedtime
- Can be used nightly

- Pay special attention to the arch of the foot
- Protective socks prevent oil stains on bedding

2. Relaxing Abdominal Massage Blend
Gentle support for nervous system and digestive calm

Ingredients:
- 2 tablespoons castor oil
- 5 drops lavender essential oil
- 3 drops bergamot essential oil
- 2 drops ylang ylang essential oil
- Small glass jar
- Hot water bottle or heating pad (optional)

Directions:
1. Combine all oils in glass jar.
2. Before bedtime, warm a small amount between palms.
3. Apply to entire abdomen in clockwise circular motions.
4. Massage gently for 5-10 minutes.
5. If desired, place hot water bottle on abdomen.
6. Practice deep breathing for 5-10 minutes.

Usage Notes:
- Best used 30-60 minutes before bedtime

- Can be used daily

- May enhance meditation practice

- Avoid bergamot if taking photosensitizing medications

NATURAL PAIN RELIEF

1. Menstrual Cramp Relief Pack

Warm application for period discomfort

Ingredients:

- ¼ cup castor oil
- 5 drops clary sage essential oil
- 3 drops marjoram essential oil
- Cotton flannel cloth
- Hot water bottle
- Old towel
- Plastic wrap

Directions:

1. Mix castor oil with essential oils.
2. Fold flannel to fit lower abdomen.
3. Pour oil mixture onto cloth until saturated but not dripping.
4. Apply cloth to lower abdomen.
5. Cover with plastic wrap.
6. Place hot water bottle on top.
7. Wrap with towel to secure.
8. Rest for 30-60 minutes.

Usage Notes:

- Begin at first sign of discomfort
- Can be repeated 2-3 times daily during menstruation
- Not for use during heavy flow days
- Store cloth in plastic container for reuse

2. Tension Headache Relief Oil

Targeted application for head and neck tension

Ingredients:
- 1 tablespoon castor oil
- 3 drops peppermint essential oil
- 2 drops lavender essential oil
- 2 drops eucalyptus essential oil
- Small glass jar

Directions:
1. Combine all oils in glass jar.
2. At first sign of tension, apply a small amount to fingertips.
3. Massage into temples, forehead, and base of skull.
4. Use gentle circular motions, applying light pressure.
5. Continue for 5-10 minutes.
6. Rest in a dark, quiet room if possible.

Usage Notes:

- Keep away from eyes

- Apply at first sign of tension for best results

- Can be repeated hourly as needed

- Store in cool, dark place

FERTILITY SUPPORT

1. Fertility-Supporting Castor Oil Pack

Traditional application to support reproductive health

Ingredients:

- ¼ cup castor oil

- 3 drops clary sage essential oil (optional)

- 100% wool or cotton flannel cloth

- Hot water bottle or heating pad

- Plastic wrap

- Old towel

- Glass container with lid for storage

Directions:

1. Mix castor oil with essential oil if using.

2. Fold flannel to fit lower abdomen.

3. Pour oil mixture onto cloth until saturated but not dripping.

4. Apply cloth to lower abdomen, covering from navel to pubic bone.

5. Cover with plastic wrap.

6. Place heating pad or hot water bottle on top.

7. Secure with towel.

8. Rest for 30-60 minutes.

9. Store cloth in glass container for future use.

Usage Notes:
- Use during follicular phase only (from end of period to ovulation)

- Do not use during menstruation, suspected pregnancy, or during two-week wait

- Most beneficial when used 3-4 times weekly for at least 3 months

- Consult healthcare provider before use if undergoing fertility treatments

References

1. *The Surprising Substances Ancient Egyptians Used to ...* https://www.smithsonianmag.com/smart-news/the-surprising-substances-ancient-egyptians-used-to-mummify-the-dead-180981568/

2. *Ayurvedic Properties of Castor Oil That Make it a Miracle Oil* https://www.ambujasolvex.com/blog/ayurvedic-properties-of-castor-oil/

3. *The Secret Magic of Castor Oil Therapy - Santa Cruz and ...* https://pointsforwellness.com/the-secret-magic-of-castor-oil-therapy-santa-cruz/

4. *Healing and Spirituality in Tanzania* https://ojs.unito.it/index.php/kervan/article/download/2872/pdf

5. *Ricinoleic Acid - an overview* https://www.sciencedirect.com/topics/agricultural-and-biological-sciences/ricinoleic-acid

6. *Castor oil: Benefits, use, and side effects* https://www.medicalnewstoday.com/articles/319844

7. *How to Use Castor Oil to Boost Your Immune System* https://www.healthydirections.com/articles/immune-health/benefits-uses-castor-oil?srsltid=AfmBOoqqeyNsEyzPPtvyOU4JvWLZIEgujujUWZYdrE6FGekoYEElb5k3

8. *An examination of the effect of castor oil packs on ...* https://www.sciencedirect.com/science/article/abs/pii/S1744388110000320

9. *5 simple ways to test the purity of castor oil at home* https://satthwa.com/blogs/carrier-oil/5-simple-ways-to-test-the-purity-of-castor-oil-at-home?srsltid=AfmBOooUtVXmG0EUd8VuQlJiReLIRuCbnU6TzP44qXqDUa6-Xl7GtR9w

10. *Castor Oil - Black Organic* https://bulknaturaloils.com/castor-oil-black-organic-s1117.html?srsltid=AfmBOoqkQsJPcj3lBTSCW-AJJbaiVRKdK7jQNQ2XhLN7A3gNg5fFkltt

11. *The Complete Guide to Storing Essential Oils* https://www.matrixaromatherapy.com/post/the-complete-guide-to-storing-essential-oils-preserving-potency-and-prolonging-shelf-life#:~:text=Proper%20storage%20in%20a%20cool,efficacy%20of%20your%20essential%20oils.

12. *Adulteration of Essential Oils: A Multitask Issue for Quality ...* https://www.ncbi.nlm.nih.gov/pmc/articles/PMC8471154/

13. *How to Use Castor Oil to Boost Your Immune System* https://www.healthydirections.com/articles/immune-healt

h/benefits-uses-castor-oil?srsltid=AfmBOor-C0CO2NmO
I7GRjnjf-mUnMegImvduqNTV45o7SLPFoIPr0Ah_

14. *How to Make and Use Castor Oil Packs* https://www.healthline.com/health/castor-oil-pack

15. *4 Laxative Recipes You Can Try at Home* https://www.healthline.com/health/digestive-health/homemade-laxative-recipes

16. *Castor Oil Packs for Natural Healing* https://jilliangreaves.com/blog/castoroilpacks

17. *Castor oil: Benefits, use, and side effects* https://www.medicalnewstoday.com/articles/319844

18. *DIY Deep Conditioning Hair Mask with Castor Oil* https://katiestewartwellness.com/2018/06/19/diy-deep-conditioning-hair-mask-with-castor-oil/

19. *Castor Oil Skin Benefits* https://epicuren.com/blogs/news/castor-oil-skin-benefits?srsltid=AfmBOooGUn9MwamWSpiG0QDE1w6ip9sWUS47gTihm5PyvVjVJqY_dUKG

20. *Can Castor Oil Be Used as Makeup Remover?* https://www.redapplelipstick.com/can-castor-oil-be-used-as-makeup-remover/

21. *Castor oil ayurveda nutrition benefits* https://www.ruhyoga.com/2020/08/12/castor-oil-ayurveda-nutrition-benefits/

22. *Balancing the Chakras Using Essential Oils* https://www.a

romaweb.com/essentialoilschakras/index.php

23. *Castor Oil Benefits and Uses* https://nikura.com/blogs/discover/castor-oil-benefits-and-uses?srsltid=AfmBOook4MLWiIYPZB2GBEFT9L-r_UGYuqz6AwD6FjdBvWkTFlp5f5dY

24. *The Transformative Power of Castor Oil Pack Rituals* https://www.shoparandi.com/blogs/news/the-transformative-power-of-castor-oil-pack-rituals?srsltid=AfmBOoq8LZQSy8K4adkGKPN9HzIS33bjQgBBEMaSwoE1R1VCGW0h7B6S

25. *Castor Oil - StatPearls* https://www.ncbi.nlm.nih.gov/books/NBK551626/

26. *Castor Oil Allergy: Risks, Side Effects, and Treatments* https://www.wyndly.com/blogs/learn/castor-oil-allergy?srsltid=AfmBOorC3AmizREkdan7DDIgHm7-lJYhMZqyyHzCl_r23ngg8hFWjfRN

27. *How to Mix Aloe Vera Gel with Oils: 9 Steps (with Pictures)* https://www.wikihow.com/Mix-Aloe-Vera-Gel-with-Oils

28. *Castor Oil: Side Effects, Uses, Dosage, Interactions, ...* https://www.rxlist.com/castor_oil/generic-drug.htm

29. *Top 5 Best Castor Oil Review in 2024* https://www.youtube.com/watch?v=5zgwOpQXY7s

30. *Important Impacts of the Shift Toward Sustainable Castor Oil* https://www.acme-hardesty.com/impact-shift-toward-sustainable-castor-oil/

31. *How to Simplify your Skincare Routine with the Oil ...* https://bottegazerowaste.com/blogs/zerowasteliving/how-to-simplify-your-zero-waste-skincare-routine-with-the-oil-cleansing-method

32. *Why Castor Oil is Trending in Clean Beauty Brands? - E r i C a r e* https://www.eri.care/blogs/news/why-castor-oil-is-trending-in-clean-beauty-brands?srsltid=AfmBOoo-4Pt074fnAH_uXXGPVjYw8RYDNfff1ozDCQ4S92Bn_k9sFZNL

33. *Castor Oil for Dogs and Cats: Benefits and Uses* https://www.earthclinic.com/pets/castor-oil-for-pets.html

34. *8 Creative Uses for Castor Oil Around the House* https://www.bobvila.com/slideshow/8-creative-uses-for-castor-oil-around-the-house-579372/

35. *Industrial Uses of Castor Oil in the Wall Paint Industry* https://girnarindustries.com/industrial-uses-of-castor-oil-in-the-wall-paint-industry/

36. *Castor Oil: Properties, Uses, and Optimization ...* https://pmc.ncbi.nlm.nih.gov/articles/PMC5015816/

37. *Castor Oil for Eczema: Effectiveness, Safety, and How to Use* https://www.healthline.com/health/eczema/castor-oil-for-eczema

38. *Castor Oil Pack* https://integrative.ca/resources/castor-oil-pack

39. *Using Castor Oil for Knee Joint Pain Re-*

lief https://www.kneepaincentersofamerica.com/blog/castor-oil-use-for-knee-joint-pain

40. *Castor Oil in Textile Industries: A Sustainable Solution for* ... https://girnarindustries.com/castor-oil-in-textile-industries-a-sustainable-solution-for-textile-manufacturing/

www.ingramcontent.com/pod-product-compliance
Lightning Source LLC
Chambersburg PA
CBHW051549020426
42333CB00016B/2173